Elements of Clinical
Research in Psychiatry

Elements of Clinical Research in Psychiatry

James E. Mitchell, M.D.
Ross D. Crosby, Ph.D.
Stephen A. Wonderlich, Ph.D.
David E. Adson, M.D.

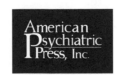

Washington, DC
London, England

Copyright © 2000 American Psychiatric Press, Inc.
ALL RIGHTS RESERVED
Manufactured in the United States of America on acid-free paper
03 02 01 00   4 3 2 1
First Edition

American Psychiatric Press, Inc.
1400 K Street, N.W., Washington, DC 20005
www.appi.org

Library of Congress Cataloging-in-Publication Data
Elements of clinical research in psychiatry / edited by James E. Mitchell ... [et al.].–1st ed.
      p.; cm.
   Includes bibliographical references and index.
   ISBN 0-88048-802-6 (alk. paper)
    1. Psychiatry–Research. I. Mitchell, James E. (James Edward), 1947-
   [DNLM: 1. Psychiatry. 2. Research–methods. WM 20 E38 2000]
   RC337.E44 2000
   616.89′007′2–dc21

                                                                99-048422

British Library Cataloguing in Publication Data
A CIP record is available from the British Library.

Contents

About the Authors

James E. Mitchell, M.D., is President and Scientific Director of the Neuropsychiatric Research Institute and Professor and Chairman of the Department of Neurosciences at the University of North Dakota School of Medicine and Health Sciences, Fargo, North Dakota.

Ross D. Crosby, Ph.D., is Director of Methodology and Statistics of the Neuropsychiatric Research Institute and Associate Professor in the Department of Neurosciences at the University of North Dakota School of Medicine and Health Sciences, Fargo, North Dakota.

Stephen A. Wonderlich, Ph.D., is Director of Clinical Research of the Neuropsychiatric Research Institute and Professor and Associate Chair in the Department of Neurosciences at the University of North Dakota School of Medicine and Health Sciences, Fargo, North Dakota.

David E. Adson, M.D., is Assistant Professor of Psychiatry at the University of Minnesota Medical School and Chair of a Medical Panel of the Institutional Review Board (IRB) at the University of Minnesota, Minneapolis, Minnesota.

Introduction

This book represents a collaboration of four individuals, all of whom are actively engaged in clinical research. James E. Mitchell, M.D., and Ross D. Crosby, Ph.D., worked together at the University of Minnesota for several years on various research projects and jointly developed and taught a course on research methodology and design for psychiatric residents. They conceived the idea for this book shortly before Mitchell moved to the University of North Dakota and the Neuropsychiatric Research Institute in Fargo, North Dakota, and recruited Crosby to come there as well. Mitchell and Crosby asked Stephen A. Wonderlich, Ph.D., already at the University of North Dakota, to become involved in the project. Wonderlich had an active research program established at the University of North Dakota and served as a mentor for investigators there. The fourth member of the group, David E. Adson, M.D., was just finishing his residency training at the University of Minnesota in Minneapolis when the project started, being retreaded from his earlier life as a family physician. He had developed an interest in clinical research and in human subjects issues and was serving on the Institutional Review Board at the University of Minnesota. He became the fourth author. He is now on the faculty at the University of Minnesota.

Although each author was responsible for drafts of individual chapters, this book represents a collaboration because we all read and made extensive revisions of one another's chapters in an effort to create a succinct, coherent, and readable text. We hope we have communicated a sense of genuine enthusiasm for clinical research and a sense of enjoyment in what we do. We do clinical research because we believe it is important, and we hope that we contribute to the welfare of psychiatric patients through our efforts. We also do clinical research because it is rewarding in several other ways, such as providing a sense of purpose; because it is intellectually stimulating and challenging; and because it gives us the opportunity to work with people whom we both enjoy and admire. We know that most practicing physicians do not imagine research to be exciting, and that is one of the main reasons many avoid it. However, it is exciting for us, and we believe it can be so for many young investigators just starting out.

James E. Mitchell, M.D.
Ross D. Crosby, Ph.D.
Stephen A. Wonderlich, Ph.D.
David E. Adson, M.D.

CHAPTER 1

Careers in Clinical Mental Health Research

Introduction

This chapter is designed to provide an introduction to and brief overview of clinical psychiatric research, and in particular to address the following questions:

1. What exactly do clinical psychiatric researchers do?

2. What decisions do individuals interested in developing careers in clinical psychiatric research need to make and when do they need to make them?

3. How does one choose an area of research and a department in which to conduct such research?

Those who read this text will be at various places along the path to developing or sustaining a research career. Some will be psychiatric residents who are considering various career options that may include clinical research. Those in this group may need help in deciding whether to take a fellowship or other additional training experience after residency, or whether to seek an appointment on a medical school faculty or in some other research setting directly. Some may be junior faculty members; their decisions about residency and fellowship versus faculty status will have already been made. Members of this group may simply want to use this book as a guide to specific areas, such as concerns about human subjects or biomedical ethics in clinical psychiatric research. Some may be medical students who are just starting their clinical rotations with a vague idea about the possibility of research. However, regardless of where individuals are on their career paths, a number of points hold true, and these are the focus of this chapter.

What Do Clinical Researchers Do?

In considering your goals as a clinical researcher, it is best to consider first what clinical researchers actually do. Clinical researchers in academic medical centers generally work in three related and overlapping spheres. The relative balance of these spheres will depend on each individual's situation, but most individuals, to some degree, participate in each:

1. Teaching (residents, medical students, fellows, at times undergraduates, and graduate students in related fields)

2. Clinical care and/or clinical administration (running a unit, running a clinic, or supervising a system of care)

3. Clinical research (in your area, but also collaborating with others in related areas)

Mentoring and Fellowships

The majority of individuals now going into biomedical research, including research in the clinical neurosciences, are those with Ph.D.'s. Furthermore, most of those who receive research grants from the federal government, serve in review groups at the National Institutes of Health, or chair those review groups are Ph.D.'s. Some think that the physician clinical researcher is becoming an endangered species.

There are several important reasons for the success of Ph.D. researchers. The single most important one is that working toward a Ph.D. requires the development and completion of a dissertation that involves a research project, and Ph.D. candidates are carefully shepherded in this process by senior faculty members. The dissertation, which occupies much of the individual's time over several years, is augmented by courses in areas such as research methodology and design, statistics, and psychometrics. Ph.D.'s are taught to think like researchers.

Medical training is not designed along these lines. Medical students and physicians are generally taught to make decisions on the basis of limited information (at times very limited), and they are taught to make these judgments quickly, since the outcome of a decision may be of extreme importance to the welfare of the patient. Although physicians can set up "experiments" to test their hypotheses (e.g., ordering liver function tests when one suspects or "hypothesizes" liver failure), the experiments are rarely of the sort required in rigorous research. Further, physicians learn very early in the course of their training that although they will need to try to keep abreast of the evolving literature in their field, they have little time and are at risk of being overwhelmed by new information. They soon discover that they can get the essence of a journal article by reading the abstract (or if time permits, perhaps the Introduction and Discussion sections). They learn that careful examination of the detailed elements of the research methodology and design in publications only slows one down, and are to be read only in unusual circumstances. Ph.D.'s are trained to be researchers: to hypothesize and to test. M.D.'s are trained to be doers: to treat, even if the experiment is flawed, and at times even if the data don't completely support the hypothesis.

As a result of such divergent training experiences, the time it takes for physicians to catch up in their research education and to develop the requisite research skills is considerable; and unfortunately, this period comes at a time when most physicians are completing their postgraduate training and attempting to launch their careers (and often trying to stay ahead of the debt payment schedule left over from medical school). This doesn't sound like a particularly propitious time in one's life to step back and to begin to learn another new field.

One way physician researchers can begin to address this disparity is to gain experience in a research environment as early as possible in their training. This may mean volunteering time (which may be hard to find) to gain research experience as a medical student and/or resident. Some medical schools now provide, and a few require, research electives for medical students for which they can receive pay or credit, and some psychiatric residencies allow potential researchers to fit into tracks for specialized research training. Other medical schools actually discourage research collaboration. Few if any clinical researchers are available to serve as mentors in some residencies, and residents in these programs are at a distinct disadvantage. The ideal situation is one in which junior residents who have an interest in clinical research are identified early and a process is established to groom them with special course work, clinical experiences, and exposure to faculty members who can mentor them.

Regardless of the method employed, one needs to get experience, as early as possible and as much as possible, with senior investigators in clinical research and to begin the process of becoming socialized into the clinical research culture.

Questions to Consider

1. How can you get some hands-on clinical psychiatry research experience? Who in your medical school (if you are a medical student) or department (if you are a resident) has an ongoing, programmatic research interest?

   Potential mentors need to be willing to accept such a role, which means being available to and supportive of the trainee, and some may not be willing to assume this responsibility. It is highly desirable for potential mentors to have an ongoing program of research (not just a single project), to have been successful in publishing their work, and to have attracted external funding (indicating that the quality of their work has been found acceptable to peers who make such funding decisions) (Yager and Burt 1994). It is also important that the potential mentor be working in an area you find interesting. The mentor need not be the most senior researcher with the most grants, since such individuals may be far too busy to offer you much in the way of help.

2. Are there courses or seminars available at your institution, or at a college or university in your area, where you can begin to learn statistics, methodology, and design? Can you get time and support from your residency director or medical student adviser for these activities?

3. Can you do a quarter or semester research elective (if a medical student)? Can you do a research elective (if a resident)?

   Unfortunately, such brief periods of time rarely give an individual the opportunity to actually complete a detailed research project. Nonetheless, the exposure can be invaluable in helping someone decide whether a research career fits for him or her.

   It is a logical extension of these points that a resident who has become interested in clinical research should carefully consider subspecialty training as a researcher. This may take the form of an emphasis on research in the fourth year, or perhaps fourth and fifth year, of residency. However, many large psychiatric research centers have training grants or internal funds to train psychiatric residents to be researchers in various fields, ranging from basic to clinical science. Some of the largest and most prestigious psychiatric residencies, such as the Western Psychiatric Institute and Clinic at the University of Pittsburgh Medical Center, Columbia-Presbyterian Medical Center, and the Intramural Program at the National Institute of Mental Health (NIMH) offer such fellowships. When considering the possibility of a fellowship, it is important to obtain information about such opportunities early in one's training and make application as early as possible.

4. How mobile are you? If it means getting the best training possible, are you willing to move (and move your family, in many cases) halfway or all the way across the country to do a one- or two-year fellowship, or are you confined to a certain geographic area?

5. How much time are you willing to devote to a research fellowship? One year? Two years? Longer, if you are training in a well-established research program and are still on the learning curve?

6. On what area do you want to focus, and with whom would you most like to train? Is this a possibility?

Teaching

Teaching can take many forms, ranging from teaching psychopathology to undergraduate medical students and psychiatric residents, to teaching clinical research to psychiatric residents and to pre- and postdoctoral fellows. Successful clinical researchers frequently find themselves in many teaching roles at various levels. It has been said that "good researchers make good teachers." Although obviously true in the sense that those who know an area in the most depth may be best able to teach it, this idea assumes that those who perform research are gifted teachers, which unfortunately is not always the case. Other parts of this book address areas of importance to teaching, such as presentations. However, academic medical educators rarely take any systematic training in how to teach, and if you want to learn to be a good teacher, you will need to seek out opportunities to learn on your own in this area.

Clinical and Administrative Work

Clinical researchers often engage in clinical and administrative work that may relate directly to the research (e.g., serving as the administrator of a clinical research unit or program or directing a clinical program that gathers research data) or that may involve activities separate from research. Put simply and obviously: the more time devoted to clinical work that doesn't result in the gathering of data for research, the less time available for your research.

This leads to an extremely important point: there is always a long list of things to do, and research often ends up being the last item on the list. Many younger investigators find that those two half-days a week that they negotiated with their chairperson to be set aside for research gradually get filled up with non-research-related clinical activities. Patients can't wait, but research can, and as a result research does not get done.

A way to manage to do research is, when possible, to have one's research and clinical populations be the same, or at least have considerable overlap; then clinical work serves one's research as well. This arrangement may be crucial in the development of a research career. Let us illustrate this point.

One of the things that many of us find fascinating about psychiatry is that when one has time to sit and discuss clinical psychiatry with colleagues, it is relatively easy to come up with a long list of interesting potential proposals for investigation in a number of clinical psychiatric populations. For example, the problem of dissociative identity disorder: it is easy to generate interesting research questions that could be addressed in this population. However, most of us don't have access to a clinical population of patients with dissociative identity disorder, and if we wanted to study such patients, it would be difficult for us to recruit them. The point is that, in order to do clinical research, one needs access to a clinical population, and this access is usually most efficiently accomplished if one runs a clinical program focused on that population. If one needs to rely on the generosity of another clinician or researcher to have access to a patient population, problems will occur.

Those who are connected with such a research population frequently get requests from outside investigators who want to administer a survey to or test a new therapy on the population. However, clinical investigators can rarely accommodate these requests, and most of this outside research, although well intended, must go undone.

Developing such a population of patients requires time, energy, and—often of most importance—administrative support. However, in addition to having access to patient populations, investigators who develop such a programmatic effort also gain a great deal of knowledge about the population and the subtleties of such patients, whereas these kinds of details may elude researchers who are only peripherally involved.

To summarize, one of the best ways to develop a clinical research program is to first develop a clinical program for the desired population, then use the population in one's research.

Habits

In thinking about establishing a research program, it is important to consider what habits younger investigators need to cultivate in order to be successful in their chosen field. These often include the following:

1. Be a good listener.

   Good researchers learn as much as they can from those around them. They learn from their patients (who in many ways are really the "experts"), from the observations of fellow staff members at all levels, and from the accumulated knowledge of other investigators in the field.

2. Read, read, read.

   The literature in any area, regardless of how finite it may seem when one first approaches it, is enormous; and in becoming a clinical researcher one must have a firm grasp, both deep and broad-based, of the field of one's inquiry, and not uncommonly several related fields as well. This is a database that will continue to change, and good clinical researchers, particularly if they hope to obtain outside funding, need to keep pace with changes in their field. The need to keep abreast of published journal articles and books will be taken for granted, and setting aside time to read the literature in one's area early in one's career is of utmost importance. But to be up to date one must also–

3. Attend national and, if possible, international meetings.

   If all that one knows about a field is what has been published in professional journals, one is at least a year out of date. The most recent information is usually presented at meetings. Established investigators also commonly circulate manuscripts to colleagues to keep them abreast of their most recent findings. Find out what the most important meetings are in your field; attend them, listen to the presentations, take notes, and study them.

4. Network.

When you begin to work in an area, it is very important to get to know the most influential people, particularly in your own geographic area, but also nationally and eventually internationally. You can find out much about which groups of investigators are doing the most important work by reading the literature and studying the work cited. Learn who these investigators are, where they are working, and what they are doing, and make an effort to meet them when they visit your area or when you encounter them at meetings. One strategy that can be employed by beginning researchers is to try to visit the laboratory or clinic of the more senior people in the field in which you would like to become established. Many senior investigators are quite open to such visits. A more senior person in your department may know these individuals personally and may provide you with a letter, e-mail, or phone call of introduction.

5. Present at meetings.

As soon as you can, submit and present scientific data at the meetings you have targeted as the most important in your field. This will allow you to obtain criticism and feedback on your work and to become known to other investigators in the field. It will also help you form the habit of organizing data and pulling together presentations in a timely fashion.

Choosing an Area of Focus

At some point, a junior investigator needs to decide on an area on which to focus. Obviously, this decision is of great importance, and it should be based on a number of factors, including the following:

1. Interest in the area and the questions that need to be asked, as well as interest in and compassion for this patient population.

If you think the area is dull, or if you dislike the patients, it is unlikely to work. If you're fascinated by the area, you are more likely to be creative in it.

2. The availability of patients and necessary equipment and/or methodology.

You're going to have trouble recruiting an adequate number of *folie à deux* cases in Walton, North Dakota, and you can't do positron-emission tomography (PET) scans in your basement.

3. Is there a niche?

A department with 10 faculty members interested in depression probably doesn't need another affective disorder researcher, but it might be a great place to train.

4. The availability of collaborators and mentors.

5. What's hot?

I mention this to discredit it. What's hot changes over time. Some investigators attempt to move their research interest to "follow the funding." What's fashionable this year may not be in two years. Put this far down on the list.

6. Areas of focus.

Areas of focus can be diagnostic groups, methodologies, or other things. For example, some researchers focus on methodology, perhaps a highly technical one like PET scanning or functional magnetic resonance imaging (fMRI), then use this technique to study more than one group of patients. Other researchers focus on a particular illness or patient group. This focus can be broad if the problem has only recently been described or has not been studied extensively (e.g., posttraumatic stress disorder), but the focus may be highly specialized in areas that have already received a great deal of attention (e.g., schizophrenia).

7. Possible hypotheses and questions.

A good rule is to sit down and elaborate these possibilities. If you find that in thinking about a clinical illness or methodology, you can come up with a variety of questions that interest you, that's a good sign.

Supportive Environment and Peer Group

One can rarely do research in isolation. A desirable situation is one in which other individuals are working in the same or related areas. It is important to work in a culture where research productivity is valued, and where recognition is given for it. The resources are also extremely important, including the availability of computers and computer time, trained research assistants, statistical consultants, and secretarial support. Many of these issues can be summarized in the following checklist:

1. How much time will you have to do research?

2. Who else in the department is doing research?

3. Where can you get advice, encouragement, and mentoring?

4. Do you have access to students or graduate students who can be hired (cheaply) to assist you?

5. Does the department have statistical support? Are there people who can enter data?

6. Are raters available who are skilled in structured clinical interviews?

7. Will you have secretarial support for your research?

8. Does the department have administrative staff who are knowledgeable about grants? Writing grant budgets? Are there people available to you who are aware of federal, state, and university or college regulations?

9. Are there others in the department who have been successful in receiving grants and who would have time to help you with grant preparation? Manuscript preparation?

10. Is there space for you to do your clinical research? Will you be using regular clinic space, or is other space available? If so, when is it available and who will pay for it?

11. Is the space available already furnished?

12. Where will you store your data? Where will you store your equipment?

13. Who will pay for equipment and for support services, such as obtaining electrocardiograms?

14. What computer access do you have? What software?

15. Who will pay for office supplies needed for you and your staff?

16. Will you be expected to pay for overhead, even if you don't have an outside grant?

17. Will the department pay for things such as rating forms, structured clinical interview forms, and other materials?

18. If laboratory testing is required, who will pay for it? Can special rates be negotiated with the hospital laboratory? Who will pay for blood drawing equipment? Is there a centrifuge to spin samples? How will the blood samples get to the laboratory?

19. How will mundane things such as phones/heat/light be provided and paid for?

20. Are sources available to pay subjects for participation or for follow-up visits if this is necessary for the experiment?

21. If medications are to be administered, are there pharmacy charges for the medications and service? Who will pay for the medication? Who will pay the setup fees? What are the dispensing fees? Will placebos be necessary?

22. Who will pay for biomedical graphics, including preparation of tables and figures for presentations and publications?

23. Who will pay to keep contracts operational on equipment such as computers and photocopy machines?

24. What are the library resources? How close is the medical library and what sort of access to it will you have? Will the department arrange to have items copied for you?

25. Is there a clinical research center available for research?

    There is a system of federally funded clinical research centers (CRCs) to which investigators can apply to use inpatient beds or conduct outpatient visits as necessary for research protocols. The costs of approved protocols are borne by the CRC. The investigator needs to negotiate specific issues, such as who will pay for pharmacy fees and laboratory costs. CRCs are extremely useful resources, but they are not always available.

Regulatory and Overview Agencies

It is important for clinical investigators early in their careers to become knowledgeable about and involved with the established university committees and oversight agencies. These include the following:

1. You will need to become very familiar with the local institutional review board (IRB) that will examine all your protocols. The IRB's prior approval will be necessary for any research involving the use of human subjects. (Chapter 8 is devoted to IRB issues). Get to know your IRB—who is on it, how often it meets, what forms are required, how often you need to submit progress reports—early in the course of your academic life.

2. Is there a university or medical school ethics committee, and if so, what sort of protocols do they want to (need to) see? Is there an area of overlap between your research efforts and what this committee considers important?

3. Many clinical researchers need to become familiar with the regulations of the pharmacy and therapeutics committee. What are the pharmacy regulations regarding the use of medications for research? Do these regulations require that investigational medication be kept in the pharmacy rather than in the investigator's office or clinic? Are there specified research pharmacists who interact with investigators, and if so, who are they?

Multiple Projects

Another point of importance in initiating a productive clinical research career is to plan for the development of several projects simultaneously. This does not evidence a lack of focus; it speaks to the fact that some projects will come to fruition and others will not, and that the time projects will take is difficult to predict. Therefore, it is important to have several going on simultaneously. Most established investigators will have two or three primary projects that occupy much of their time, but will have several add-on projects going as well, often projects they are doing collaboratively. The best advice is to start as many projects as you comfortably can and to collaborate with and help others (who will help you) on related projects they are pursuing. The days are over when people retreated to their laboratory or isolated clinic space to do research. Most research of real consequence is done in groups working together on multiple projects proceeding simultaneously.

Summary

It's hoped that this chapter has served as a useful introduction to the area of clinical psychiatry research. The task of developing such a career may seem daunting, but it can also be challenging and energizing. Clinical research can be an exciting field, and in the chapters that follow we hope you will find useful information and advice.

CHAPTER 2

Research Design

Research Questions

One of the first steps in the development of a research design is the selection of a research question. The research question should be of interest not only to the individual researcher but also to some recognized segment of the psychiatric community. Often the research is a replication and/or extension of a previous project. The research question should also have some practical or theoretical significance, adding to our existing knowledge or contributing meaningfully to the field. Equally important, the research must be feasible to perform. Consideration should be given to the costs of conducting the study. One cost is of course monetary, but other costs, such as time and effort, must also be considered and may turn out to be deciding factors. Finally, ethical considerations, such as the withholding of treatment or the invasion of privacy, must also be considered in the selection of a research problem.

It is useful to develop a precise statement of the research question. It serves to delineate in broad terms what the study is about, as well as what it is not about. This statement, which may be in either descriptive or question form, should include a clear and concise statement summarizing the key factors or variables involved in the study. The following are examples of statements of research problems that provide adequate focus and direction:

Descriptive form: A study of the effects of naltrexone on alcohol consumption in adult outpatients being treated for alcohol dependence

Question form: What motivational and personality factors are associated with outpatient treatment retention in female adolescents with bulimia nervosa?

The statement of the research question provides a general focus and direction for the research study. However, it does not include all the specific information necessary for conducting the study. Consider the second example above. We know that the study focuses in general on the relationship between motivation, personality, and treatment retention. However, a number of important questions remain unanswered—for example: What personality factors are being examined? How are they measured? What is the expected relationship between a given personality factor and treatment retention?

Research Hypotheses

Research hypotheses provide the specificity and direction for these types of questions. A research hypothesis is a precise statement about the relationship between two or more variables. The hypothesis should be brief, concise, and, most important, testable. It should also be stated in such a manner that the results of the study serve to sustain or refute the hypothesis. The research hypothesis often contains an operational definition of how the construct in question is to be measured. Following are some examples of testable research hypotheses.

The following two hypotheses are directional hypotheses, since they specify the direction of association or difference:

A negative relationship exists between Avoidant total scores on the Wisconsin Personality Inventory and the number of outpatient treatment visits completed by female adolescents with bulimia nervosa.

The percent of positive alcohol Breathalyzer tests in adult outpatients being treated for alcohol dependence is lower for subjects given naltrexone than for subjects given placebo.

In contrast, nondirectional hypotheses predict a difference or an association but do not specify its direction or pattern. The following is a nondirectional hypothesis:

Scores on the Obsessive-Compulsive scale of the Wisconsin Personality Inventory will differ between female adolescent outpatients with bulimia nervosa and those with anorexia nervosa.

Whether a hypothesis is stated in directional or nondirectional form is determined by the expected results. Often, previous research or theory has established an anticipated direction for the relationship and thus led to directional hypotheses. In contrast, exploratory studies often use nondirectional hypotheses.

Types of Research Designs

The statement of the research question and the subsequent research hypotheses will help to determine the type of research design used. Three broad classes of research designs can be identified: experimental designs, quasi-experimental designs, and observational designs. The characteristic features of each class, along with relevant examples, appear below.

Experimental Designs

Experimental designs are distinguished by three essential features:

Manipulation. In all experimental designs, one or more variables—referred to as *independent variables*—are deliberately manipulated or varied by the researcher to determine their effects upon another variable, referred to as the *dependent variable*. A researcher, for example, may manipulate the medication being received (e.g., naltrexone vs. placebo) in order to observe its effects on alcohol consumption.

Randomization of individuals. The purpose of randomization is to control or balance out the effects of any extraneous variables. In the example above, a third variable, the severity of alcohol dependence, may be related to a patient's response to naltrexone. When patients are assigned randomly to naltrexone or placebo, the effects of dependence severity on alcohol consumption are balanced out across the treatments; any differences in dependence severity between the two groups at the beginning of the study are due to random variation and not the treatment per se.

Control or comparison group. In psychiatric treatment outcome research, commonly used control groups are a no-treatment group, a waiting-list group, a placebo group, and a standard-care group.

Quasi-Experimental Designs

Quasi-experimental designs (Campbell and Stanley 1963), like experimental designs, involve the manipulation of an independent variable. In contrast to experimental designs, however, quasi-experimental research involves the use of intact groups of subjects, rather than subjects assigned at random to experimental treatments. Randomization may be involved; however, random assignment is performed at the group level rather than at the individual level. Quasi-experimental designs are frequently used in psychiatric research when it is impractical to assign individuals randomly to treatment conditions. For example, a researcher investigating a new outpatient treatment for depression may randomly assign entire treatment clinics to experimental or control conditions.

Types of Experimental/Quasi-Experimental Designs

Three general types of experimental/quasi-experimental designs can be identified:

Within-subjects designs. The distinguishing feature of within-subjects designs is that subjects are exposed to multiple treatments or interventions. There are several types of such designs; two are discussed here:

• Two-period crossover design. In this design, half of the subjects receive treatment A first, followed by treatment B. The remaining subjects receive treatment B first, followed by treatment A. The order of treatments is typically randomized. This design is frequently used to compare an active medication to placebo.
• Latin square design. This design uses incomplete counterbalancing to control for the effects of sequence. Rather than including all possible treatment sequences, the Latin square design selects a subset of sequences such that each treatment appears once in each ordinal position. A 3×3 Latin square is shown in Figure 2–1. Note that all groups receive all three treat-

Group 1	A	B	C
Group 2	B	C	A
Group 3	C	A	B

Figure 2–1. A 3×3 Latin square.

ments and that each treatment appears only once in each ordinal position. Comparisons between treatments are thus made within subjects.

Between-subjects designs.   In contrast to within-subjects designs, subjects involved in between-subjects designs are exposed to only one intervention or treatment. Comparisons between treatments are thus made across groups rather than within subjects. Examples of between-subjects designs follow:

- Pretest-posttest control group design. As the name implies, two groups are assessed before an intervention is made. The intervention is then applied to one group, and postintervention assessments are again performed for both groups. If individual subjects are randomized to groups, this is a true experimental design. On the other hand, if no randomization is used, or if groups are randomized to treatment or control conditions, the design is quasi-experimental. Often, quasi-experimental designs use matching to equate nonrandomized groups on variables that may affect outcome.
- Randomized block design. In this variation of the pretest-posttest control group design, subjects are grouped in blocks on the basis of some confounding variable and randomized into treatment within these blocks. An example is a study examining the effects of a new treatment versus standard treatment for depression. Because we suspect that gender may affect response to treatment, we block subjects by gender and randomize within genders to new or standard treatment. The advantage of the randomized block design is that the effects of the confounding variable on outcome can be statistically removed, allowing for a more powerful design.
- Randomized clinical trial (RCT) design. RCTs assess the efficacy of a treatment by comparing outcomes in a group of patients receiving a test treatment with those in a comparable group of patients receiving a control treatment; patients in both groups are enrolled, randomized, treated, and followed over the same period. The RCT is considered the current scientific standard for establishing the efficacy of psychiatric treatment.

Single-case designs.   Single-case designs are used to assess the effects of an experimental intervention on individual subjects. There are several types:

- A-B-A-B reversal design. In this design, a baseline assessment period (A) is used to establish a stable pattern of behavior. Then an experimental intervention is applied, and the effects of this intervention are determined in a second observational period (B). After a stable pattern of behavior is observed, the intervention is withdrawn. The effects of the withdrawal are again observed (A) until a stable pattern emerges. This reversal pattern can be repeated a number of times to establish a clear association between intervention and behavior change.

- Alternating treatments design. In this design, treatments (or interventions) are alternated on successive days or sessions. This sequence is repeated over several days (or sessions), and differences in the behaviors observed within each treatment period are compared.

- Multiple baseline design. A multiple baseline across behaviors involves an initial baseline assessment of several behaviors. After a stable pattern is observed, an intervention is applied to a specific behavior. The effects of this intervention are observed for both the target and nontarget behaviors. Once a stable pattern is observed, the intervention can then be applied to another behavior. This sequence can be repeated until the intervention is applied in sequence to all behaviors of interest. The multiple baseline design can also be applied across multiple subjects or across multiple settings.

Choosing an Experimental/Quasi-Experimental Design

A variety of factors can be considered in deciding between within-subjects, between-subjects, and single-case designs.

One obvious factor is the *availability of subjects*. Clearly, single-case studies can be done with very few subjects. Typically, within-subjects studies require fewer subjects than between-subjects studies, since in the former design each subject serves as his or her own control.

Another factor is the *nature of the treatments*. Many single-case designs (e.g., A-B-A-B reversal, alternating treatments) and most within-subjects designs require treatments that are relatively transient and reversible. Treatments such as psychotherapy that result in permanent changes are not suitable for these designs.

A third factor is the possibility of *subject attrition* or *dropout*. Within-subjects designs are much more compromised by subject attrition than are between-subjects designs. Typically, if subjects in within-subjects studies terminate before receiving all treatments, their data are not usable.

A fourth factor is the possibility of *carryover effects* from multiple treatments. In within-subjects studies, there is the possibility that the effects of one treatment may persist in some fashion at the time of measurement of another treatment. Examples of carryover effects include learning, sensitization, and pharmacological carryover from medications. These carryover effects are likely to bias the comparisons between treatments in within-subjects designs. If carryover is likely, a between-subjects design is a better choice.

The fifth and final factor is the issue of *generalizability of findings*. Clearly, the results of single-case designs are least generalizable because of the very limited sample size. In general, the results from within-subjects studies are more generalizable, but the confounds and biases from multiple treatments may limit their generalizability in comparison to between-subjects designs.

Observational Designs

The third broad class of research designs is *observational designs*. Their characteristic feature is that they involve measurement without the manipulation of independent variables. One example is survey research, in which the relationship between variables is studied in its natural setting. Another example is epidemiological studies that examine the relationship between risk factors and disease. Research within this class can be either cross-sectional, in which data are collected at a single point in time, or longitudinal, in which data are collected across multiple time points.

Two common observational designs in epidemiological research are the case control study and the cohort study.

Case control study. The case control study design is a retrospective one, in which groups with and without the particular disease of interest are selected. These disease/no-disease groups are then assessed to determine retrospectively their exposure to various risk factors. A higher rate of exposure to a risk factor in the disease group than in the no-disease group is indicative of a possible causal link between risk factor and disease.

Cohort study. The cohort study design is a prospective one, in which groups with and without a risk factor are selected. These groups are then followed prospectively to determine the percentage of each group that develops the disease. A higher disease rate in the group with the risk factor is indicative of a possible causal link between risk factor and disease.

Internal and External Validity

Kerlinger (1986) has suggested that the purpose of a research design is twofold: first, to provide answers to research questions, and second, to control variance. The first of these purposes is relatively straightforward. Good research designs provide a means for obtaining usable results as well as a basis for understanding and interpreting these results.

The second purpose of research design—controlling variance—involves two related issues. First, research is conducted in order to demonstrate a relationship, or shared variance, between two or more variables. For example, an experiment is designed to demonstrate that the intervention, the independent variable, caused some effect or change in the dependent variable. The second aspect of controlling variance involves potential confounding variables. Sound experimental designs control for the effects of other variables that may be related to the dependent variable and eliminate these variables as possible explanations for the findings. The reader is referred to the previous discussion of randomization as a method for controlling the variance of a confounding variable (the section in this chapter titled "Randomization of individuals").

How do we evaluate the adequacy of a research design? How do we determine to what extent the research design provides clear answers to our research questions? Campbell and Stanley (1963) have suggested that research designs can be evaluated in terms of two properties: internal validity and external validity.

Internal Validity

Internal validity is to the extent to which we are able to make inferences about the relationship between variables. It relates to our ability to make logical conclusions from the results of our study. Consider the previously mentioned study of naltrexone in the treatment of alcohol dependence. Suppose it is found that the percentage of Breathalyzer tests positive for alcohol is lower for patients treated with naltrexone than for patients treated with placebo. Internal validity is the extent to which we are confident that the medication, and not some other factor, accounts for the differences between the two groups.

A variety of factors pose threats to internal validity. These factors are considered in detail elsewhere (Campbell and Stanley 1963; Cook and Campbell 1979) and will be only briefly highlighted here.

- One threat to internal validity is *history,* unanticipated events occurring during the course of a study that may affect the dependent variable. Research designs without adequate control or comparison groups are particularly susceptible to historical confounds.
- Another threat is *selection bias,* distortion due to differences in the manner in which subjects were initially selected. Quasi-experimental designs, which in-

volve preexisting groups, frequently do not control for selection bias. Therefore, these groups may differ in ways unrelated to the intervention that may
account for the differences in outcome measures. The primary method for
controlling selection bias is the random assignment of individuals.

- A third threat is *information bias,* distortion due to systematic measurement
  or misclassification of subjects. This bias is particularly important in retrospective studies, where factors such as recall and diagnostic surveillance
  may be substantially different in patient and control groups.

In general, it can be stated that threats to internal validity are best controlled in experimental designs, somewhat less controlled in quasi-experimental
designs, and least controlled in observational designs. One should not conclude from this, however, that all designs within a given class are equivalent.
A careful consideration of the threats to internal validity identified by Campbell and Stanley (1963) when researchers are planning a research design will
help to identify potential confounds and serve to strengthen the overall design. Further, it should be pointed out that each type of design has its place in
psychiatric research. Experimental designs are best suited for hypothesis
testing. Unfortunately, many research problems are not amenable to controlled experimental study. In those cases, quasi-experimental designs often
are a viable alternative. Quasi-experimental designs can be seen as providing
a balance between practicality and experimental rigor. Observational designs are particularly useful for descriptive research and can be helpful in
generating hypotheses in exploratory research.

External Validity

The other criterion by which we evaluate the adequacy of a research design is
external validity, the extent to which we are able to generalize findings about
the relationship between variables to a larger target population. Let us consider again the study of naltrexone in the treatment of alcohol dependence.
External validity relates to the extent to which we are able to generalize these
results to other settings and to other patients. Again, there are threats to this
type of validity:

- One obvious threat is the *reactive effects* of the experiment itself. Subjects
  know that they are participating in an experiment. This knowledge may
  cause them to react in ways different from the reactions of subjects who
  are exposed to the intervention but who are not a part of an experiment.
  This has become known as the Hawthorne effect.

- Another threat is *multiple treatment interference:* the carryover effects in subjects receiving multiple treatments may not be generalizable to subjects receiving single treatments.
- A third threat is the *manner in which the treatment interacts with the selection of subjects or with the setting in which the research takes place.* Consider the vast amount of randomized clinical medication trials currently being sponsored by pharmaceutical companies. The interaction of treatment with selection and setting relates to the extent to which the findings of these trials can be generalized to patients other than study volunteers or settings other than a structured research facility.

Improving External Validity

What can be done to increase the external validity of your research design? Cook and Campbell (1979) offer three suggestions.

- The first method is to randomly sample from the population of interest. This will ensure that the sample is representative of the population within known limits of sampling error. Unfortunately, this is frequently impractical in psychiatric research.
- A second method is to deliberately sample for heterogeneity. This will help to ensure that a wide range of subjects is represented in the design.
- A third method is referred to as *impressionistic modal sampling.* It involves identifying *before the research begins* the types of persons or settings to which one wants to generalize, then selecting at least one instance of each class that is "impressionistically similar" to that class mode.

CHAPTER 3

Measurement

Introduction

There is an important distinction between the concepts of measurement and statistics. *Measurement* is the process of assigning numbers to represent some property, such as the quantity or quality of an object. Examples of measurement include using inches to represent distance, IQ scores to represent intelligence, and integers to represent gender (e.g., 1 = male, 2 = female). In contrast, *statistics* is a collection of methods for summarizing, displaying, or analyzing numerical data, often for decision making. Graphs, descriptive statistics (e.g., mean, standard deviation), correlations, and tests of differences (e.g., *t* tests, analyses of variance [ANOVAs]) are all examples of statistical methods. Measurement provides the numbers that are summarized and/or analyzed by statistics. The distinction is important, because the adequacy of the measurement process, assessed in terms of the reliability and validity of the measure, ultimately affects the conclusions that are drawn from the statistical analyses. The use of inadequate measures often leads to inappropriate or erroneous conclusions.

In this chapter we provide a general overview of the issues relating to measurement. Included is a discussion of the various ways in which numbers are used to represent properties–the so called levels of measurement. Also considered are topics pertaining to the adequacy of measurement techniques, including a discussion of reliability and validity. Finally, the validity of diagnostic measures is considered. Readers interested in obtaining a more

23

comprehensive consideration of measurement are referred to Nunnally (1967) or Anastasi (1982).

Levels of Measurement

Measurement involves the process of assigning numbers to represent some property or construct. Numbers can be used in a variety of ways. Some numbers, for example, may represent a quantity, like pounds or inches; other numbers may represent a particular quality or category, like positive or negative. Four distinct ways in which numbers can be assigned to represent a property have been identified (Stevens 1951): nominal, ordinal, interval, and ratio. These so-called levels of measurement are important for two reasons:

- First, the level of measurement provides information about the relationship between individual elements to which numbers are assigned. For example: Is element A greater than element B? Is the distance between element A and element B greater than the distance between element B and element C?
- Second, the level of measurement frequently dictates the appropriate statistical methods for summarizing and/or analyzing the data.

Nominal Scale

A *nominal* scale uses numbers to represent some qualitative class or category. Examples include using numbers to represent gender (e.g., 1 = male, 2 = female) or marital status (1 = never married, 2 = married, 3 = divorced, 4 = widowed, 5 = other). The numbers themselves have no inherent meaning; they connote no particular order or direction. The numbers in a nominal scale may be changed (e.g., 1 = female, 2 = male) without reflecting any change in the properties of the elements themselves.

Ordinal Scale

An *ordinal* scale uses numbers to reflect a rank ordering of elements in relation to some property. However, the numbers in an ordinal scale do not express the true magnitude of the elements in relation to this property. Further, ordinal numbers cannot be used to express the distance between elements, merely their relative ranking. House addresses are an example of an ordinal scale. We know that a house with the address 2200 is farther down the street than the house with the address 2150. However, we cannot conclude that the distance between the houses at 2150 and 2200 is the same as the distance between the houses at 3150 and 3200. Another common example of ordinal scales is the use of Likert-type items, such as the one in Figure 3–1. Although on a Likert-type scale a −2 indicates stronger agreement than −1, the difference between −2 and −1 may not be the same as the difference between −1 and 0.

Interval Scale

An interval scale uses numbers to reflect some quantity. As with the ordinal scale, the relative order of the numbers in an interval scale is important. In addition, however, the relative *distance* between elements in an interval scale is important.

Interval scales typically have a zero point. The distinguishing feature of the interval scale is that the location of the zero point is arbitrary and does not reflect the complete absence of some property. Examples of interval scales include the Celsius and Fahrenheit temperature scales. Each scale has a different unit of measure and a different zero point, yet in both scales the distance between temperatures is meaningful and informative. Also note that in neither scale does the zero point reflect an absolute absence of temperature (i.e., 0° F does not mean that there is no temperature).

Another example of an interval scale is IQ scores. Again, the distance between scores in meaningful and informative, but an IQ of zero does not represent the absence of intelligence.

Interval scales (and ratio scales as described below) are often referred to as continuous. However, this does not necessarily imply that all numerical values are possible on these scales.

Ratio Scale

A ratio scale has all the properties of an interval scale plus a fixed and nonarbitrary zero point reflecting the complete absence of some property. Examples of ratio scales include height in inches, weight in pounds, and age in years. Only when a scale has an absolute zero point does the ratio of num-

Strongly agree	Agree	Uncertain	Disagree	Strongly disagree
−2	−1	0	1	2

Figure 3–1.   Likert-type scale.

bers become informative. For example, it is correct to conclude that 20 pounds is twice as heavy as 10 pounds. Contrast this to an interval scale. It would not be correct, for example, to conclude that 20° F is twice as much temperature as 10° F. The difference is that 0° F does not reflect the absence of temperature, whereas 0 pounds does reflect the absence of weight.

Scales of Measurement and Statistical Methods

Any of the ordinary arithmetic operations (addition, subtraction, multiplication, and division) may be applied to interval and ratio scales, and the result will maintain information about the magnitudes of the elements in relation to the underlying property. Classical measurement theory (e.g., Stevens 1951) dictates that arithmetic operations are not appropriate for nominal or ordinal scales. However, there are instances in which such operations can be informative. As an example, consider a sample of subjects who are assigned a 1 if male and a 0 if female. In this case, the mean of the variable representing gender is equivalent to the proportion of the sample that is male.

The discussion by Hays (1973) on levels of measurement and corresponding statistical methods (pp. 87–90) is useful to consider. Hays contends that there are many instances when the level of measurement may not reach the level required by the statistical technique, yet that technique may be quite adequate for the intended purpose. Any statistical method designed for numerical scores can be applied to numerical data in which the interval-scale level of measurement is not met, provided that the purely mathematical/statistical requirements of the methods are met. Reiterating Lord's (1953) axiom: "The numbers don't remember where they came from, they always behave just the same way, regardless" (p. 751). It is the role of the experimenter to exercise appropriate caution in the use and interpretation of these results. This issue will be considered in more detail in the following chapters.

Evaluating the Adequacy of Measurement: Reliability and Validity

As pointed out previously, the adequacy of the measurement process has a marked effect on the conclusions that are ultimately drawn from the data. The adequacy of a measure can be evaluated in terms of two basic properties of measurement: reliability and validity.

Reliability

Reliability is the extent to which a measure yields the same results on successive trials. A reliable measure is one that produces consistent results when applied in the same manner. Some measures, such as length and weight, are extremely reliable, producing nearly identical results across repeated applications. Other measures, such as measures of personality or psychiatric symptoms—constructs of great interest to clinical psychiatric researchers—are much more variable. Factors that may influence reliability include characteristics of the test taker (e.g., motivation or concentration), the evaluator (e.g., appearance, interpersonal style), the testing situation (e.g., physical environment, distractions), or the test itself (e.g., mode of administration).

Indices that measure reliability typically range from 0.00 to 1.00; values closer to 1.00 indicate greater reliability. The reliability of a measure can be determined in a variety of ways, discussed next.

Internal consistency. Measures of internal consistency, such as Cronbach's (1951) alpha or Kuder and Richardson's (1937) KR-20, provide an index of the interrelatedness of items within a test. Larger values indicate higher average interitem correlation. In general, measures of internal consistency, such as alpha, will increase as the number of items increases (Green et al. 1977). This is because additional items are likely to include slightly different aspects of the construct being measured. Thus, other things being equal, we would expect higher alphas from a scale containing 30 items than from a comparable scale containing only 10 items.

Split-half reliability. Split-half reliability involves randomly dividing a test into halves and determining the correlation between scores on each half. Split-half reliability, like measures of internal consistency, is based on the intercorrelation of items. In fact, Nunnally (1967) considers the corrected split-half correlation to be an estimate of the coefficient alpha.

Alternate-form reliability. Alternate-form reliability is the correlation between scores on two different (but equivalent) forms of the same measure. The advantage to alternate forms is that they minimize the problem of a test taker's remembering how he or she responded on a previous administration. The greatest drawback to alternate-form reliability is the difficulties associated with developing equivalent forms.

Test-retest reliability. Test-retest reliability is the correlation between scores of individuals on the same test obtained at two different points in time. Test-retest reliability is typically referred to as the stability of a measure over time. What is the optimal interval for obtaining test-retest data? The answer depends in large part on the nature of the trait being measured. Some traits, such as personality characteristics, are considered to be relatively stable. Consequently, a test-retest interval of several months would be appropriate. In comparison, depressive symptomatology is known to fluctuate substantially over time. Therefore, a much shorter test-retest interval (e.g., 1 week) would be appropriate in that case. The key to selecting an appropriate test-retest interval is choosing an interval that is 1) short enough that observed differences between testings are not likely to be due to actual changes in the trait being measured and 2) long enough that the test taker is not responding merely on the basis of memory.

Reliability: Other Comments

The most commonly used indices of reliability are measures of internal consistency (particularly alpha) and test-retest reliability. The specifics of the test, including the construct being measured, the practicalities of collecting retest data, and the expressed purpose of the test will ultimately determine which form or forms of reliability are most suitable in a given circumstance.

How reliable should a test be? Although the easy answer would be "as reliable as possible," the practical limitations of clinical research rarely allow the use of a test with perfect reliability. Consequently, some general guidelines are in order. As a general rule of thumb, a reliability of .80 can be used as a minimal acceptable level. This value should be lowered slightly (e.g., .75) for tests with fewer than 10 items and raised slightly (e.g., .85) for tests with more than 25 items. Keep in mind that these are only general guidelines that may need to be modified in some circumstances.

What are the effects of reliability on repeated observations? Wainer and Thissen (1996) conducted a simulation study in which they generated scores for subjects on two parallel forms, assuming that the examinees did not change between administrations. The test scores were normally distributed, and scores were generated for tests ranging in reliability from 0.00 (i.e., random) to 0.94. Table 3–1 summarizes the observed differences in scores between testings.

Wainer and Thissen (1996) noted that a test that has a reliability of 0.40 is better than a random number, "but not much" (p. 23). Even with a reli-

Table 3–1. Differences in retest scores as a function of test reliability

Test reliability	% of tests differing by more than		
	0.5 SD	1.0 SD	1.5 SD
0.00	72%	48%	29%
0.40	65%	36%	17%
0.60	58%	26%	9%
0.80	43%	11%	2%
0.90	26%	3%	0.1%
0.94	15%	0.4%	0.0%

Note. SD = standard deviation.

ability of 0.80, 43% of the scores vary by as much as a half standard deviation, and 11% vary by as much as a full standard deviation. (See Chapter 5, section titled "Standard deviation," for a description of standard deviation). If we are interested in measuring change as a function of some treatment, and if the changes we would expect are on the order of a half standard deviation, then this reliability is clearly unacceptable. The table provided by Wainer and Thissen (1996, p. 24), along with the reliability of a particular measure, can be used to estimate the number of individuals in a given study who will change by a given amount due to chance alone. These estimates can provide broad guidelines for minimal acceptable levels of reliability.

Validity

Validity is the extent to which a given measure actually represents the intended property. Reliability is a prerequisite for validity. However, demonstrating reliability does not ensure validity. Consider the following example: two testers are hired to measure the head circumferences for a group of 30 individuals. After both testers have measured all 30 people, it is discovered that the testers never disagreed by more than $\frac{1}{16}$ of an inch on any individual. Is the measure reliable? Without question! Clearly the results were extremely consistent across testers. Is the measure valid? This question cannot be answered without asking "Valid for what?" If the measure is intended to represent hat size, the validity is undoubtedly extremely high. On the other hand, there would probably be little evidence to support the validity of this measure as an indicator of IQ. Thus, validity is always evaluated in terms of the intended purpose of the measure.

Forms of Validity

Face validity.   Face validity refers to the extent to which the test actually measures what it appears to measure at face value. Tests with high face validity are typically obvious and direct. In contrast, tests with low face validity are typically indirect, and the purposes of the test may not be readily apparent to the test takers. Although face validity is not a prerequisite for other forms of validity discussed below, test takers may be more receptive and less defensive when taking a test with high face validity than one with low face validity (Anastasi 1982).

Content validity.   Content validity refers to the extent to which a measure includes a representative domain of the content related to the construct being measured. For example, a measure of depression with high content validity might include items on mood, activities, weight loss, sleep patterns, energy level, feelings of worthlessness, concentration, thoughts of death, and somatic complaints. The better the measure reflects the content domain of the construct, the greater the content validity. Content validity is often established by using experts in the field and/or professional literature to identify the relevant content domains. Items are then generated to represent these content areas. The correspondence between items and content domains can then be verified by requiring raters to sort items into the appropriate content domains.

Construct validity.   Construct validity refers to the extent to which evidence is provided that the intended construct is actually being measured.

One way in which construct validity can be established is by demonstrating agreement (typically a correlation) between the measure in question and another measure of the same trait. This is referred to as *convergent validity*. For example, evidence for the convergent validity (and therefore the construct validity) of a new measure of depression can be established by demonstrating a strong positive correlation between that measure and other previously validated measures of depression, such as the Beck Depression Inventory (Beck et al. 1961).

Another means of establishing construct validity is by demonstrating a lack of relationship between the measure in question and measures of other conceptually unrelated traits. This is referred to as *discriminant validity*. For example, depression is not conceptually related to IQ. Therefore, a strong correlation between this measure of depression and IQ scores would raise questions about the construct validity of the measure.

Criterion-related validity. Criterion-related validity is the extent to which a measure relates to some external criterion (e.g., behavior). A distinction is made between criteria obtained at the same time as the measure (referred to as *concurrent validity*) and criteria obtained at some point after the measure (referred to as *predictive validity*). For example, the predictive validity of a depression measure could be demonstrated by showing a positive correlation between depression scores and prospective suicide attempts.

Diagnostic validity: sensitivity and specificity. Many types of measures are designed to provide a qualitative binary classification: present/absent, positive/negative, and so forth. One example is a measure designed to provide a definitive psychiatric diagnosis, such as major depressive disorder. The methods involved in establishing the validity of diagnostic instruments are somewhat different from the methods used for conventional quantitative measures. As these methods are particularly relevant to many clinical research applications, they deserve some consideration here.

The validity of diagnostic instruments is always established in relation to some established gold standard: a new psychiatric diagnostic instrument is evaluated in relation to an existing structured psychiatric interview such as the Structured Clinical Interview for DSM-III-R (SCID) (Spitzer et al. 1992); a new laboratory assay is evaluated against an existing laboratory assay. Consider the following example. A new test of depression provides a diagnosis for major depressive disorder (MDD): present (referred to as a positive test) or absent (negative test). The diagnostic efficiency of this new test is compared with an existing gold-standard diagnostic test, which also provides a diagnosis for MDD: present (referred to as a positive case) or absent (negative case). A group of individuals are given both tests. The results can be presented in a 2 × 2 table displaying test instrument diagnosis (positive/negative) by gold-standard diagnosis (positive/negative). An example is presented in Table 3–2. The letters A–D represent the frequency of individuals in each cell.

Table 3–2. Diagnostic validity: sensitivity and specificity

Test	Gold standard	
	Positive case	**Negative case**
Positive test	A	B
Negative test	C	D

Sensitivity = A/(A + C)
Specificity = D/(B + D)

Diagnostic validity (frequently referred to as diagnostic efficiency) can be represented by two properties:

- *Sensitivity* refers to the percentage of all positive cases correctly identified by the test instrument: $A/(A + C)$. In the present example, a sensitive depression measure correctly identifies the majority of individuals that actually have depression (as determined by the gold standard).
- *Specificity* refers to the percentage of all negative cases correctly ruled out by the test instrument: $D/(B + D)$. A specific depression measure correctly produces a negative test for the majority of individuals that do not have depression (again as determined by the gold standard).

A good diagnostic instrument has both high sensitivity and high specificity. Stated differently, high diagnostic efficiency involves correctly identifying a majority of the positive cases and correctly ruling out a majority of negative cases. What are acceptable levels of sensitivity and specificity? Acceptable levels depend on a variety of factors, including currently available diagnostic instruments, the quality of the gold standard, the costs of false-positive and false-negative error, and the purposes of the test. Typically, purely diagnostic instruments have comparable levels of sensitivity and specificity. On the other hand, screening instruments typically have much higher levels of sensitivity (e.g., >0.90) than of specificity.

CHAPTER 4

Assessment

Introduction

In clinical research, the properties of measurement described in the previous chapter become critical because they guide the researcher in selecting measurement strategies that will be used in the assessment of the research subject. The *assessment* of a subject often refers to a broader and more comprehensive concept than simple measurement or testing, which may be elements of the assessment procedure (Goldstein and Hersen 1990). When planning the assessment phase in research, the researcher first needs to consider how he or she will measure the behaviors and/or features of the subjects to be examined in the study. This assessment process should be carefully informed by the hypotheses underlying the study.

Imagine, for example, that Dr. X wants to test the idea that playing video games reduces hallucinatory activity in schizophrenic individuals. What behaviors or characteristics of the subjects does she need to assess?

- First, she needs to assess potential subjects to demonstrate that they indeed have schizophrenia.
- Second, she may have secondary hypotheses that motivate her to measure other characteristics of the subjects (e.g., social adjustment, occupational functioning, comorbid psychopathology), and if so, she needs to derive a strategy for measuring each of these characteristics.

- Third, she may want to assess whether the treatment intervention is applied appropriately—find a strategy that verifies that the video game treatment is delivered in the manner in which she believes it should be delivered. This is sometimes called a validity check.
- Fourth, she needs to measure hallucinatory activity, the dependent variable.

In each of these instances, she needs to select measures for each facet of the assessment that are reliable and valid. She also needs to select a battery of instruments that can be administered in a finite period of time, so as not to demand too much of her subjects.

Characteristics of Measures

Kazdin (1992) has delineated a number of ways in which assessment measures used in clinical research may vary. These include the following:

- *Global versus specific.* Does the measure quantify very broad domains of functioning (e.g., life satisfaction or emotional state) or more specific domains (e.g., body size estimation, severity of depression)?
- *Public versus private behavior.* Is the measurement designed to assess public overt behaviors (e.g., compulsive buying) or private behaviors (e.g., negative self-statements)?
- *Stable versus transient.* Does the measure attempt to assess a transitory phenomenon (e.g., affective states) or more stable characteristics (e.g., intelligence)?
- *Direct versus indirect.* Is the subject aware that the assessment is taking place (e.g., semistructured interview) or unaware that the assessment is actually occurring (e.g., unobtrusive measure of behavior on the inpatient ward)?
- *Breadth of domain.* Does the measure assess a variety of constructs (e.g., the full range of DSM personality disorders) or does the measure assess a single construct (e.g., hypnotic susceptibility)?
- *Format.* Is the level of depression in a depressed subject, for example, being measured by a semistructured interview, a clinical interview, a paper-and-pencil self-report inventory, or an outside informant (e.g., spouse)?

When one considers the almost endless number of behaviors or clinical conditions that can be measured and the various ways in which assessment measures can differ, the number of measurement strategies can become overwhelming. That is why researchers need to carefully consider what, according to the research hypotheses, needs to be measured, then to pay careful attention to the psychometric qualities of the assessment devices that may be chosen. Otherwise, the research may become lost in the morass of available measures for an endless number of constructs.

Modes of Assessment

The number of particular behaviors, traits, or other human characteristics that can be measured is limited only by the interests and creativity of the researcher. However, there are several well-established modes of assessment, or methods of measurement, that are often used in clinical research in psychiatry. These modes of assessment have been reviewed previously (Dennis et al. 1992; Hersen and Bellack 1981; Kazdin 1992) and are only briefly mentioned here.

Global Ratings

Global ratings refer to judgments made by an *observer* regarding global characteristics or level of functioning of the self or subject. Often, these are measured on a 5- or 7-point scale, commonly referred to as a Likert-type rating scale. Such a scale is typically anchored by two extreme behavioral descriptors that reflect the range of functioning on the dimension being assessed. Figure 4–1 shows this type of scale, on which the rater is asked to assess how much a subject's anxiety impaired his or her ability to function at work.

Although such rating scales typically refer to *general* subject capabilities or functions, more precise and specific behavioral ratings could also be made. The value of using such rating scales to assess global constructs of human behavior is that the measure can be applied across diagnostic groups and various treatment studies in a standardized manner. This may be particularly important in large-scale clinical outcome studies, which are becoming in-

No impact, work performance unaffected	1	2	3	4	5	6	7	Extreme impact, unable to work

Figure 4–1. Likert-type global rating scale.

creasingly common in psychiatry. For example, the Global Assessment of Functioning (GAF) scale used in DSM-IV (American Psychiatric Association 1994) allows a very generic, but useful, measurement of overall patient functioning to be assessed across a wide variety of patients and conditions. Another example, the Personality Assessment Form (PAF) (Elkin et al. 1985) relies on clinician's ratings of patients' personality functioning that has a general correspondence to each of the DSM personality disorder diagnoses. The PAF was used in the National Collaborative Study on the Treatment of Depression (Elkin et al. 1985) and is an example of a fairly well-defined set of rating scales. Other commonly used clinical rating scales for general psychopathology include the Nurse's Observation Scale for Inpatient Evaluation (NOSIE-30; Honigfeld and Klett 1965) and the Ward Behavior Inventory (Burdock et al. 1968). These scales rely on ratings of patient behavior by nurses or psychiatric aides on a series of items assessing behaviors such as cooperativeness, appearance, communication, and aggressive episodes.

The advantage of such global rating scales is that they reduce a significant amount of complex behavioral information to a relatively simple measurement; the risk is that such measurement may be too simple. For example, if a researcher wants to measure the efficacy of a new treatment for depression and relies on therapist's global rating of how well the patient responded to the treatment as a sole outcome measure, he or she might obtain a simplistic and potentially erroneous measurement. Another possible problem with global rating scales is what has been termed "rater drift" (Reid 1970). Because these scales often do not provide highly operationalized criteria to guide the ratings, a rater's application of the scales may vary across time and situation, depending on numerous factors influencing the individual rater. In addition, different raters may interpret the scale differently, which also poses threats to the reliability and validity of the measure. However, in spite of these potential limitations, global rating scales often provide a useful measurement of meaningful constructs that may be a valuable method as a part of an overall assessment strategy.

Self-Report Questionnaires and Tests

Whereas global rating scales provide a measurement of a *rater's* perception of a research subject, self-report measures allow the *subjects* to provide information regarding their own behavior, subjective experience, or perceptions of the environment. Such scales typically ask subjects to rate or judge how they view various aspects of their own personality, cognition, affect, or overt behavior, as well as their perceptions about other people or things.

In part because of the historical value placed on the subjective experience of the subject, and also because of the ease of administering such measures, self-report questionnaires abound in behavioral research. Such measures assess a wide variety of constructs, which can be easily measured across numerous situations. Some of the better-known self-report measures of psychopathology in behavioral research include the Minnesota Multiphasic Personality Inventory (MMPI; Hathaway and McKinley 1943), the Beck Depression Inventory (BDI; Beck et al. 1961), and the Hopkins Symptom Checklist–90 (SCL-90; Derogatis and Cleary 1977), but there are other tests that assess a wide variety of other constructs, such as family functioning, cognition, affect, and eating behavior–to mention only a few of the research areas where self-report measures are used.

The major problems associated with self-report measures relate to the subjective nature of the ratings by the subject. In other words, for various reasons, subjects' ratings of their thoughts, feelings, or behavior, or the behavior of others, may be spurious. Two kinds of distortion are frequently mentioned in referring to self-report measures. The first, typically called *response style,* refers to a particular strategy the subject may use in completing the questionnaire, a strategy that has little to do with the content of the items and that consequently distorts the results (Lanyon and Goldstein 1971). For example, if the questionnaire relies on a true-false format, a subject may alternate true and false responses throughout the questionnaire, with no apparent relationship to the content of the item. Similarly, if the response format of the questionnaire asks subjects to endorse one of three response options, a subject may select option 2 for most or all items, regardless of content. Clearly, such a style of responding, which is unrelated to the content of the items, invalidates the measure.

Another source of distortion in such self-report questionnaires is the presence of response sets. Here, subjects endorse items in a specific way because they wish to present themselves in a particular manner on the questionnaire (Lanyon and Goldstein 1971). For example, some individuals may distort their responding because they wish to present themselves in a socially desirable manner, and minimize any problems they might have. This may be seen when subjects deny ever having thoughts about suicide, when in fact they do, if they believe the researcher may judge them negatively for reporting such thoughts. On the other hand, some individuals may attempt to present themselves as ill if they believe that appearing too well adjusted or healthy may not be in their best interest. For example, if schizophrenic individuals want to remain in the hospital and fear that the absence of psychotic symptomatology may result in a discharge from the hospital, they may present themselves as highly disturbed, with an overestimation of the frequency or severity of their psychotic symptoms on the self-report measure.

A final source of distortion in self-report measures is that certain state effects related to acute psychopathology may significantly distort subjects' ratings of their long-term behavioral functioning. For example, individuals who are in the midst of an acute depression may rate certain features of their personality or environment much more negatively than they would after their depression has resolved. Distortions in the perception of "stable" characteristics such as personality (e.g., Hirschfeld et al. 1983) or perceptions of early family life (Lewinsohn and Rosenbaum 1987) have been reported in the literature and highlight the potential risk of state-related effects of psychopathology on self-report measures.

Clinical Interviews, Structured Interviews, and Semistructured Interviews

If the psychiatric researcher wants to use psychiatric diagnoses as either independent or dependent variables, there is consensus that the diagnoses should be made through an interviewing process rather than self-report questionnaires (Goldstein and Hersen 1990). This is due in part to the previously mentioned response sets and potential for distortion associated with self-report questionnaires. Although not totally free of the potential for distortion, interviews allow for more intensive, precise, and clinically informed questioning regarding the behaviors associated with a particular diagnostic criterion than do self-report questionnaires. Thus, self-report measures are frequently used as screening measures and are followed up with some type of interview to further clarify the diagnostic status of the subject (Hunt et al. 1984; Zimmerman 1994).

However, psychiatric interviews have their own problems. For example, if researchers use routine *clinical* interviews to confirm diagnoses, they may gain information directly from the interview questioning as well as indirectly from chart notes, information from outside informants, and data from any other source that they think would help them in making a diagnosis. However, such an approach may lead two clinicians, both conducting a clinical interview of the same patient, to arrive at a different diagnostic outcome because of the wide variety of sources of information they may receive and use. This phenomenon, referred to as *information variance* (Endicott and Spitzer 1978), is considered a major threat to reliability in interviewing strategies. Another threat to reliable interviewing is what is referred to as *criterion variance*. This term refers to the tendency of two clinicians to use different inclusion and exclusion criteria when establishing a diagnosis. For research purposes, interviews are best viewed as a tool to give clinicians information that will help them make a diagnosis based on a clearly defined set of diagnostic criteria. If the criteria are not explicitly operationalized and detailed, clinicians may construct their own intuitive and highly variable diagnostic hunches, based on their personal beliefs about a psychiatric disorder.

In an effort to control the effects of information variance, psychiatric researchers have increasingly turned to structured and semistructured interviews. These interviews differ from the routine clinical interview because every interviewer is required to ask the same set of diagnostic questions, or probes, to evaluate the diagnostic criteria. Requiring an interviewer to assess the same domains of psychopathology and use the same questions to assess these domains reduces information variance and enhances reliability.

Furthermore, structured and semistructured interviews are typically tied to a specific set of diagnostic criteria, a method that reduces criterion variance. For example, one popular structured interview, the Schedule for Affective Disorders and Schizophrenia (SADS; Endicott and Spitzer 1978), is linked to a particular set of diagnostic criteria called the Research Diagnostic Criteria. Similarly, the Structured Clinical Interview for DSM-IV (Spitzer et al. 1992) is linked to the diagnostic criteria outlined in DSM-IV. When a structured or semistructured interview is completed and diagnoses are made, the researcher can be somewhat assured that the information has been derived from the same general source and that the criteria used to make the diagnosis are objective, preestablished, and explicitly linked to the interview itself. Of course, this process is not perfect, and two interviewers could use these procedures and still reach different diagnoses for the same patient. The evidence suggests, however, that this approach significantly enhances reliability when compared with routine clinical interviewing strategies (Wiens 1990).

Behavioral Assessment of Overt Behavior

Behavioral assessment refers to a collection of procedures that together represent a major advance in measurement strategies in behavioral sciences over the last three decades (Goldstein and Hersen 1990). Goldstein and Hersen suggested that behavioral assessment developed as a reaction to a number of factors, including the following:

- Problems with the reliability and validity of the earlier DSM-I and DSM-II diagnostic schemes
- Concerns about the indirect relationship between traditional psychological testing and treatment planning

- The increasing impact of behavior therapy as a treatment modality
- Parallel developments in the field of diagnosis that emphasized greater precision and accountability

Behavioral assessment refers to a broad range of procedures that includes behaviorally explicit interviews, ratings, self-report instruments, self-monitoring procedures, and the observation of specific overt behaviors. However, in contrast to more traditional psychometric theory, each of these procedures identifies specific observable behaviors rather than measuring abstract latent constructs. Thus, behavioral assessment relies heavily on procedures that allow for the specific identification and counting of specific behavioral phenomena. Early behavioral assessment strategies emphasized measurement of overt behaviors, such as hair pulling, head banging, time spent sleeping, and aggressive behavior. However, as behavior therapy broadened its scope to begin to include cognitive and affective variables, behavioral assessment also began to use self-report measures and interviews to identify cognitive and emotional variables. However, behavioral assessment of overt behavior continues to be an indispensable assessment strategy.

Behavioral assessment of overt behavior refers to observing direct samples of the behavior, rather than using self-report questionnaires, interviews, or global rating scales of abstract constructs. Such an approach relies on a careful operational definition of the behavior in question, which allows an observer to count or tally when it occurs. For example, if a researcher wanted to develop a measure of hyperactive behavior in children, he or she might measure the number of times that a child leaves his or her desk in the classroom setting, thus defining hyperactivity, at least in part, as *out-of-desk behavior*. Similarly, a researcher wishing to develop a measure of trichotillomania might define such behavior as any occurrence of the subject's hand touching the hair on his or her head. Operational definitions of depression might include the amount of time spent in bed by the depressed individual. It can be seen that these measures do not assess a global multifaceted construct but instead focus on specific measurable behaviors thought to be of relevance to a part of the construct being studied.

Typically, behavior therapists rely on behavioral assessment to develop behaviorally oriented treatment strategies. Once a sound operational definition and measurement system has been developed for a particular behavior, behavioral clinicians might conduct a functional analysis, in which they would identify the antecedents and the consequences of the behavior. For example, they may notice that a hyperactive child leaves his or her desk whenever another child walks past, and that this usually results in the teacher's attending to the hyperactive child. Treatment may then evolve directly from these observations by modifying antecedents and consequences of out-of-desk behavior. Alternatively, the trichotillomanic individual may engage in hair pulling only when watching television or engaged in some other form of self-stimulatory activity, which may again lead to helpful environmental interventions.

One of the greatest problems associated with behavioral assessment of overt behavior has to do with the representativeness of the assessment. Put differently, is the sample of behavior collected representative of the typical domain of behaviors exhibited by the individual across time and situations? For example, suppose researchers want to assess the frequency of hair-pulling behavior by a child with trichotillomania. They agree to go to the child's school and observe the child over the lunch hour every day for 1 week. Will this observation schedule provide an accurate and valid assessment of the child's hair-pulling behavior? Perhaps the child is less likely to pull hair while eating. This observation schedule could severely distort the behavioral assessment of the child's hair-pulling behavior. Consequently, sound behavioral assessment must be based on repeated sampling across various times and situations to give a comprehensive assessment of the conditions associated with the behavior.

Another problem associated with behavioral assessments is that frequently such assessments take place in artificial situations, such as laboratory settings, which provide a high degree of methodological control. However, the representativeness of the behavior in such an environment may be minimal—a phenomenon that poses significant problems for this method of assessment. For example, the alcohol consumption of subjects in a contrived laboratory situation or the binge-eating behavior of a bulimic individual in a feeding laboratory may not represent the subjects' typical drinking and eating behaviors outside the laboratory. Thus, every effort should be made in behavioral assessment to enhance the representativeness and generalizability of the assessment from the laboratory to the environment in which it naturally occurs.

Psychobiological Assessment, Laboratory Tests, and Brain Imaging

With the greater emphasis on biological factors and biological therapies in psychiatry, there has been increased interest in the assessment of biological processes associated with various forms of psychopathology (Morihisa et al. 1996). With increasing sophistication in the technology of biological assessment, the number of assessment strategies available to the clinical researcher has grown substantially in the last few decades. For example, simple screening procedures used for detecting physical disease may include variables that can fit into a particular research protocol (e.g., complete blood count [CBC], thyroid function tests, electrocardiogram [ECG]). Also, other more specific laboratory tests—such as lumbar punctures with examination of obtained cerebral spinal fluid, urine and blood toxicology determinations, and laboratory evaluation for environmental toxins— may all be included in research protocols. The electroencephalogram (EEG) also has a long history of use in behavioral research and can be used in a wide variety of studies to examine brain electrical activity.

Research on biological markers in psychiatry continues with various types of neuroendocrine challenge tests, including the dexamethasone suppression test, the thyrotropin-releasing-factor (TRF) stimulation test, and the corticotropin-releasing-hormone stimulation test. Recently, brain imaging has become a valuable way of directly assessing the functioning of the human brain. Functional brain-imaging techniques include computerized electroencephalography, evoked-potential mapping, positron-emission tomography, single photon emission computed tomography, and regional cerebral blood flow studies. Structural brain-imaging techniques such as magnetic resonance imaging and computed tomography have begun to provide new perspectives in information on the structural brain abnormalities associated with various forms of psychopathology.

These assessment strategies may provide numerous benefits to research assessment protocols. For example, unlike self-report measures, the measurements obtained from psychobiological assessment cannot be consciously distorted or manipulated by the subject. Similarly, such measures provide much more specific assessment of a particular process that is not attainable with global rating scales. Despite these advantages, sole reliance on psychobiological assessment as a measure of a particular construct may be quite limiting. For example, determining the metabolic activity in the brains of depressed people in a study examining correlates of depression does not preclude the need for self-report of depression by the subject. Furthermore, it is important for the psychiatric researcher to remember that these advances in psychobiological assessment do not ensure quality research. If the fundamental research design in which such assessment procedures are used is flawed, the conclusions from the study will also be flawed, despite the highly technological and expensive assessment procedures. Therefore, it is important for the researcher to remember that the use of highly technological assessment strategies does not guarantee good science.

Principle of Multiple Measurement

In some psychiatric research studies, a single mode of assessment may adequately measure the constructs for the hypothesis being tested. For example, if a researcher wants to test the idea that a drug will reduce hair pulling in trichotillomania, a simple behavioral measure of hair pulling may be sufficient. Similarly, if a researcher hypothesizes that the sleep EEG tracings of family members of depressed probands will be different from the tracings for family members of control subjects, a single EEG measurement can adequately test the hypothesis.

However, behavior is often complex and multifaceted. Depression, for example, may have some features that are best assessed by self-report (e.g., subjective sense of sadness, low self-esteem), others best assessed by behavioral observation (e.g., slow motor behavior, excessive sleep), and still others best assessed by psychobiological modes of assessment (e.g., EEG tracings). Consequently, the nature of human behavior and psychopathology often requires multifaceted assessment of basic theoretical constructs.

Furthermore, although the researcher might like to believe that the modes of assessment for a particular construct will covary, they often do not. For example, suppose a researcher is testing a hypothesis that a new psychotherapy effectively treats bulimia nervosa. It is possible to imagine that a bulimic individual may self-report a decreased amount of food consumed during binge-eating episodes. However, careful behavioral assessment in a laboratory may reveal that there is no change in the amount of food consumed during binge-eating episodes. By assessing complex behavioral constructs through multiple channels of measurement, the researcher gains both a more accurate assessment and a more comprehensive understanding of the nature of the construct being studied.

Finally, another reason for using multiple modes of assessment is the problems associated with what is often called *method variance.* Suppose that a researcher is attempting to examine the relationship between a wide variety of affective states (e.g., sadness, anxiety, anger, happiness). In order to test the covariance of these mood states, the researcher administers a self-report measure for each one of the constructs. It is possible that the scores on these measures will covary, not because the constructs themselves covary, but because all the measurement is conducted within the self-report mode of assessment. Perhaps subjects endorse more items on all scales because all the scales happen to be self-report format. If other indicators of these affective states, measured by other modes of assessment (e.g., observer rating scales, behavioral observation), were included, the covariance might be substantially different.

A Hypothesis-Driven Approach to Assessment

Psychiatric research is most often an effort to test an idea. When this idea, or hypothesis, is clearly delineated, it informs and guides the selection of assessment devices. In theory-driven research, the researcher asks the question, What do I need to measure in order to adequately and precisely test my hypothesis? Supporting questions are these: Does the hypothesis require measurement of a construct in only a single mode of assessment? On the other hand, are there theoretical reasons or empirical findings suggesting that the researcher should measure the constructs of interest across multiple modes? If so, which modes should be selected and why? In some research settings, these decisions will be determined by the logistics of the research setting. For example, if the researcher is conducting epidemiological surveys with a national representative sample of respondents, the self-report or interview modality will obviously be used to measure the constructs of interest. Similarly, if the researcher wants to assess changes in depression levels across time in developmentally disabled individuals, he or she may have to rely on global ratings completed by informants or behavioral observation because of the subjects' inability to complete self-report forms adequately. Although such logistical and practical factors may substantially influence measurement in a study, the researcher should also carefully consider how the hypotheses and associated theory should influence assessment strategies.

CHAPTER 5

Descriptive Statistics

Introduction

We begin this chapter with an example that will help delineate the meaning of the term *statistics* and differentiate two major types of statistical techniques, *descriptive* and *inferential* statistics.

A psychiatrist wants to learn more about the patients he is treating. He decides to perform structured diagnostic interviews at intake on all patients he sees in his clinic over the course of 1 year. He records these data, along with measures of depression and anxiety at intake and at all subsequent visits. At the end of 1 year, he has a database of 85 patients. He now is ready to analyze the data with statistics.

Statistics

Statistics is a collection of methods for summarizing, displaying, and analyzing numerical data, often for the purposes of decision making.

Descriptive statistics are methods for organizing, summarizing, and communicating data. The purpose of descriptive statistics is to characterize and delineate a specific data set; there is no attempt to make inferences beyond the available data. Thus the psychiatrist in the example above may calculate the mean number of Axis I (DSM-IV; American Psychiatric Association 1994) diagnoses, the percentage of patients with a mood disorder, or the correlation of depression and anxiety scores at intake, or he may create a frequency distribution of anxiety disorders. All these are examples of de scriptive statistics because they describe or summarize some aspect of the data.

Inferential statistics, in contrast, are methods of analyzing data in order to arrive at conclusions extending beyond the immediate data. Inferential statistics are typically used as a basis for decision making or hypothesis testing. In the example above, the psychiatrist may wish to know whether female patients have significantly fewer Axis I diagnoses than male patients, or whether patients with a somatization disorder have significantly poorer outcomes in terms of reduction of depression and anxiety symptoms than do patients without a somatization disorder. These are examples that rely on inferential statistics, because the conclusions that the psychiatrist will make extend beyond the immediate sample of patients that has been measured.

The purpose of this chapter is to provide a general overview of descriptive statistics. First, methods for describing a "typical" score in a distribution, so-called *measures of central tendency,* are considered. Next, methods for describing the spread of a distribution, referred to as *measures of dispersion,* are highlighted. Finally, techniques for characterizing the *relative location* of individual scores are considered. Inferential statistics are considered in the following chapter.

Descriptive Statistics

Measures of Central Tendency

One of the most straightforward ways of characterizing a distribution of numerical scores is in terms of an "average" or "typical" score. Measures of central tendency provide a summary statistic that is representative of the distribution as a whole. Consider the following distribution of 10 test scores:

$$3, 4, 5, 5, 5, 6, 6, 7, 9, 10$$

What number would best describe and characterize the distribution as a whole?

Mode. One possibility would be to describe the distribution in terms of the *most frequently occurring* score. This is referred to as the *mode.* The mode of the distribution above is 5, since that score occurs more frequently (three times) than any other score. The use of the mode to describe a distribution has several advantages. The mode is easy to calculate and interpret. It may also be used to describe any distribution, regardless of whether the measure is categorical or numerical. However, the mode also has certain disadvantages. A distribution may have more than one mode. A distribution with two modes is referred to as *bimodal*. In distributions with more than one mode, the mode loses it effectiveness as an indicator of a "typical" score. Also, for continuous measures with an infinite number of possible values, the mode is generally uninformative.

Median. Another possibility for characterizing a set of scores is by using the midpoint of the distribution: the point at or below which 50% of the cases fall. This is referred to as the *median*. The median is determined by arranging scores in order from lowest to highest. For distributions with an odd number (N) of scores, the median is the middlemost score (i.e., the score at $[(N + 1)/2]$ in order); for distributions with an even number of scores, the median is the score midway between the scores at $[N/2]$ and $[(N/2) + 1]$ in order. The median for the distribution of the 10 test scores in the preceding section is 5.5, since that is the midpoint between 5 (the fifth ordered score) and 6 (the sixth ordered score). The median is generally considered to be more informative about the "typical" score than is the mode. In contrast to the mean (described below), the median is less sensitive to extreme scores. As a result, the median is typically used to describe distributions with a few extremely large (or extremely small) scores, such as a distribution of annual incomes. The major disadvantage of the median is that it does not take into account the value of every score. This can be demonstrated by changing the score of 10, in the previously listed distribution of test scores, to 20. The median (5.5) remains unchanged.

Mean. A third method for describing a distribution of scores is to state it in terms of the arithmetic average. This is referred to as the *mean*. The mean is calculated by summing the scores and dividing by the number of scores. The mean for the distribution of 10 test scores above is 6.0 (60/10). The mean can be thought of as the "balance point" of a distribution. As any number in the distribution is changed, the value of the mean changes as well. Thus, the mean, unlike the median and mode, takes into account the value of every score. Another unique feature of the mean is that the signed deviations of scores around the mean always sum to 0. This can be demonstrated by subtracting the mean from each score and maintaining the sign ($\pm$) indicating whether the score is above or below the mean. The sum of those deviations will always be 0.

Characteristics of the mode, the median, and the mean. If you were trying to guess a score picked at random from a distribution, which score should you choose? If you wanted to be right most often, you should guess the mode. Since the mode is the most frequently occurring score, guessing the mode will provide you the best likelihood of hitting the number on the nose. If instead you wanted to make the smallest amount of error, irrespective of sign, you should guess the median. Since the median is the middlemost point, it is closest on average to all the scores. Finally, if you were interested in balancing errors, so that on average you were neither above nor below the actual number, then you should choose the mean. Recall that the sum of the signed deviations around the mean is always 0.

Measures of Dispersion

Measures of dispersion describe the spread, or extent of differences, among scores in a distribution. Stated differently, measures of dispersion indicate the tendency for scores to depart from central tendency. Just as measures of central tendency can be thought of as "best guesses" in a given distribution, measures of dispersion can be thought of as an indicator of the extent to which these measures of central tendency are inadequate to describe a single score.

Range. One measure of dispersion is the *range*. The range is the difference between the largest and the smallest scores in the distribution. The advantages of the range include its ease of computation and its simplicity of interpretation. The chief disadvantage of the range is that it is based on only two scores: the minimum and maximum. Changing any of the other scores, as long as they do not exceed the minimum and maximum bounds, will have no effect on the range. As a consequence, other measures of dispersion, such as the variance and standard deviation, are generally more informative.

Variance. The *variance* is the average squared deviation from the mean. Put differently, the variance tells us the average squared numeric distance between a subject's score on a measure and the group's average on that measure. The variance is calculated by subtracting the group mean from each individual observation, squaring the difference, summing those differences across all scores, and dividing by the number of scores. The deviations around the mean are squared because, as shown previously, the signed deviations around the mean always sum to 0. As an example, the variance of the 10 test scores referred to previously is shown in Figure 5–1.

The variance, like the mean, is sensitive to the relative value of all scores and is influenced by extreme scores. The variance will be 0 when all scores have the same value, and it will become larger as the scores become more disparate from each other and the mean. The major disadvantage of the variance is that it expresses dispersion in terms of squared units of measurement. For example, if measurements of height are made in inches, the mean is also expressed in terms of inches. However, the variance is expressed in terms of squared inches. As a consequence, it is difficult to interpret the variance without converting back to the original measurement units. This provides the rationale for the final measure of dispersion, the standard deviation.

Standard deviation. The *standard deviation* is the square root of the variance. The standard deviation of the 10 test scores in the example given earlier is the square root of the variance (4.2), which is 2.049. The standard deviation shares all the properties of the variance: it takes into account all scores and is sensitive to extreme scores. In addition, however, the standard deviation expresses dispersion in terms of the original measurement units. But how does one make sense of this number? As will be seen in the following chapter, if a particular distribution is normally distributed, the approximate percentage of cases between any two scores can be obtained from a table of normal values. However, this technique is not particularly useful for distributions that are markedly different from the normal distribution. A more useful method for

Score	Mean	Difference	Difference squared
3	6	-3	9
4	6	-2	4
5	6	-1	1
5	6	-1	1
5	6	-1	1
6	6	0	0
6	6	0	0
7	6	1	1
9	6	3	9
10	6	4	16

Sum of differences squared: 42
Variance = 42/10 = 4.2

Figure 5-1. Calculation of the variance of 10 sample test scores.

interpreting standard deviations is provided by Chebychef's theorem. This theorem states that for *any* distribution, regardless of shape or size, *at least* $[1 - (1/k^2)]\%$ of the scores will lie within k standard deviations of the mean. This provides extremely useful information for any value of k above 1. Values for k and $[1/k^2)]$ are presented in Table 5–1.

From Table 5–1, we find that for *any* distribution, regardless of its degree of normality or overall shape, at least 56% of all scores fall within 1.5 standard deviations of the mean, 75% within 2 standard deviations, and 89% within 3 standard deviations. These figures can be used as general guidelines for evaluating how typical (or atypical) a given score is compared with the distribution as a whole.

Calculating variance and standard deviation. The question often arises as to why the variance and standard deviation are calculated in terms of deviations around the mean. The answer is that the average squared deviation

Table 5–1. Values of k and $[1-(1/k^2)]$ for Chebychef's theorem

k	$1-(1/k^2)$
1.1	.17
1.2	.31
1.3	.41
1.4	.49
1.5	.56
1.6	.61
1.7	.65
1.8	.69
1.9	.72
2.0	.75
2.2	.79
2.4	.83
2.6	.85
2.8	.87
3.0	.89
3.5	.92
4.0	.94
4.5	.95
5.0	.96

(and therefore the variance and standard deviation) is smallest when calculated around the mean. This property accounts for the fact that the mean and standard deviation provide the basis for a variety of the statistical tests described in the following chapter (e.g., t test, analysis of variance [ANOVA], correlation).

Other Descriptive Statistics

Two other descriptive statistics are often useful for communicating features about the shape of a distribution.

Skew. The *skew* of a distribution is an index of symmetry. A distribution is symmetrical only if it is possible to divide the distribution into two mirror-image halves. The skew of a distribution is calculated as 3 times the difference between the mean and the median, divided by the standard deviation. Thus, the skew of the 10 test scores discussed previously,

$$3, 4, 5, 5, 5, 6, 6, 7, 9, 10$$

   is

$$[3(6.0 - 5.5)]/2.049 = .732$$

The sign and magnitude of the skew indicate the direction and degree (respectively) of the asymmetry. A skew of 0 indicates a symmetrical distribution. A positive skew indicates more extreme values on the right (i.e., positive) tail of the distribution; a negative skew indicates more extreme values on the left (i.e., negative) tail of the distribution. The skew of a distribution often provides information about the relative location of the mean, the median, and the mode. This is shown in Figure 5–2.

A symmetric unimodal distribution (i.e., skew = 0) will result in identical values for all three measures of central tendency. In a unimodal positively skewed distribution, the mean is greater than median, which in turn is greater than the mode. The converse is true for a unimodal negatively skewed distribution. The relative position of the three measures of central tendency in skewed distributions is accounted for by the fact that the mean, as the balance point of a distribution, is sensitive to extreme scores.

Kurtosis. The *kurtosis* of a distribution refers to the steepness of its peaks when displayed graphically. A distribution with observations clustering more around the mode is referred to as *leptokurtic*. A flatter, more evenly distributed curve is referred to as *platykurtic*. This is illustrated in Figure 5–3.

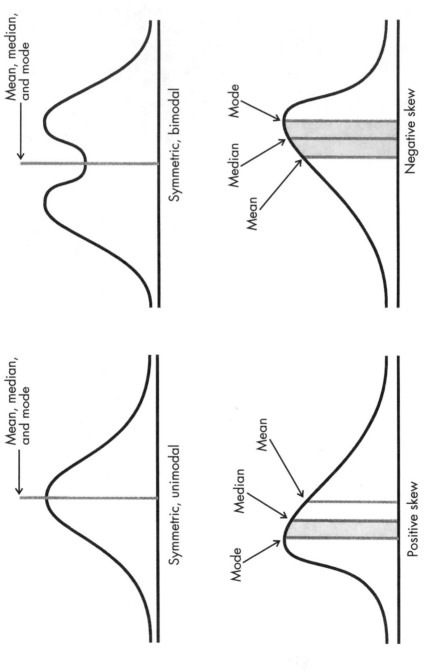

Figure 5–2. Symmetric and skewed distributions.

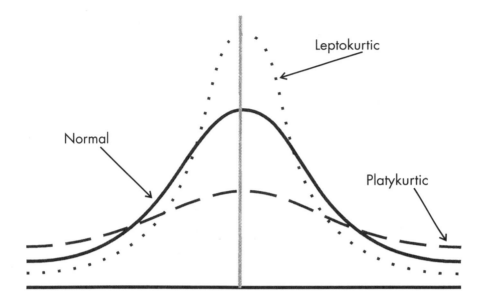

Figure 5–3. Kurtosis.

Skew and kurtosis in evaluating distribution. Skew and kurtosis are often used as a basis for determining whether a given distribution is distributed normally. Many of the inferential statistics (e.g., ANOVA, *t* test) described in the following chapter assume that the observations are distributed normally. Skew and kurtosis thus provide a means of evaluating this assumption statistically. The normal curve is considered in more detail in the following chapter.

Relative Location of Individual Scores

Consider the following example. A psychiatric patient is given two clinical tests, one for anxiety and one for depression. The results of the tests, along with information about the performance of other patients in the clinic on these tests, are presented in Figure 5–4. (Note on the figure: z-scores and t-scores are discussed at the end of this chapter.)

A psychiatrist wants to evaluate these scores in two ways: first, to compare the patient's anxiety and depression scores with each other as a means of identifying which is the more problematic condition; and second, to compare these scores with the scores of other patients in the clinic. How can these comparisons best be made?

It is clear that the raw scores from the two tests are not directly comparable. Both the maximum total scores and the mean scores for all clinic patients

Scores and statistics	Test	
	Anxiety	Depression
Maximum total score	35	60
Mean (other clinical patients)	20	40
SD (other clinical patients)	4	10
Patient's total score	28	45
Patient's percentile rank	95th	70th
Patient's z-score	2.0	0.5
Patient's t-score	70	55

Figure 5–4. Relative location of individual scores: a patient's scores from two clinical tests.

are markedly different on the two tests. The patient's score must be evaluated in relation to the scores of other patients on this test. This can be accomplished in at least three ways.

Percentile rank. The patient's score can be represented in terms of the percentage of all scores that are at or below the score achieved by the patient. This is referred to as the *percentile rank*. On the anxiety test, 95% of the clinic patients scored at or below the patient's score of 28. In contrast, on the depression test, only 70% of the clinic patients scored at or below the patient's score of 45. This suggests that the patient's anxiety score is more elevated than the depression score. Although the percentile rank expresses the percentage of scores at or below a particular point, it is not informative about the overall spread of scores.

Z-scores. Another way to express the relative location of individual scores is in terms of *z-scores*. A z-score is a measure of how many standard deviations a given score is above or below the mean of the scores for the sample from which the subject came. For example, a z-score of 1.0 would indicate a score one standard deviation above the mean, and a z-score of –2.5 would indicate a score $2\frac{1}{2}$ standard deviations below the mean. Z-scores are computed by subtracting the mean of the distribution from the individual score and dividing the result by the standard deviation. The patient's score of 2.0 on the anxiety test, compared to 0.5 on the depression test, indicates that, although both scores are greater than the mean for clinical patients, the former is more elevated.

A z-score is generally considered to provide more information about the relative standing of a score than do percentile ranks. Consider that both of the terms used to calculate a z-score, the mean and standard deviation, are influenced by the values of *every* score. In contrast, changing individual scores in a distribution will not necessarily change the percentile rank for a given score.

Z-scores are linear transformations of some original distribution. If all the original scores are converted into z-scores, the distribution of z-scores will always have a mean of 0 and a standard deviation of 1. Z-scores change the "unit" of measurement, but do not change the shape or the mathematical form of the distribution. This can be confirmed by graphing the distributions of raw scores and z-scores; they will look identical except for the unit of measurement. It can also be shown that the correlation (see the following chapter) between raw scores and z-scores is 1.0 for any distribution.

T-scores. Many psychological and psychiatric tests are based on *t-scores*. T-scores, like z-scores, are standardized scores that allow the comparison of scores across distributions. Whereas the distribution of z-scores has a mean of 0 and a standard deviation of 1, t-scores have a mean of 50 and a standard deviation of 10. A t-score of 60, which is equivalent to a z-score of 1.0, indicates a score one standard deviation above the mean. T-scores are calculated by multiplying the z-scores by 10 and adding 50. To avoid negative numbers, t-scores are often used rather than z-scores. T-scores, like z-scores, change the unit of measurement but not the form of the distribution.

CHAPTER 6

Inferential Statistics

Introduction

In this chapter we introduce three topics that are essential background for a discussion of inferential statistics: sampling, probability, and normal distribution. Once these have been considered, three types of inferential statistics will be highlighted: point estimation, interval estimation, and hypothesis testing.

Inferential Statistics and Sampling

Inferential statistics are methods of analyzing data to arrive at conclusions extending beyond the immediate data. Contrast this to *descriptive statistics* (see previous chapter), whose purpose is merely to describe or summarize a specific data set.

Consider the following example: a researcher believes that a new screening test may help in the detection of bulimia nervosa. The researcher gives the test to a group of 100 patients with a previous diagnosis of bulimia nervosa and a comparable group of 100 control subjects without bulimia nervosa. The researcher then compares the groups on the basis of their test scores. Is it the intention of the researcher simply to demonstrate that these two groups are different, judging from the test? Clearly not! If the researcher were only interested in demonstrating that the groups themselves were different, no tests of statistical significance would be necessary. It would suffice to simply show that the groups scored differently on the test, no matter how large or small that difference actually was. In this case, the researcher is interested in making conclusions that extend beyond the groups actually being measured. The statistical comparisons the researcher performs address the question of whether the differences observed between the groups support the conclusion that the populations from which they were drawn are different—that is, whether there are differences between patients with bulimia nervosa and comparable subjects without bulimia nervosa.

The previous example illustrates the framework for inferential statistics: conclusions about some larger group are made on the basis of a subset of that group. The larger group is referred to as a *population*. A population is the totality of units under study. It is the group or collection of observations to which a researcher ultimately hopes to apply research conclusions. In psychiatry, we often attempt to make conclusions that will generalize to a much larger patient population than we actually measure in a given study. Summary characteristics, such as means and standard deviations, that are used to describe populations are called *population parameters*. A *sample* is a part or a subset of the population. Summary characteristics that are used to describe samples are referred to as *sample statistics*. Thus, inferential statistics is the process of drawing inferences about population parameters by using sample statistics.

Probability

Probability plays an integral role in inferential statistics by providing a basis for making inferences about a population by using characteristics of the sample. As such, it is important to consider various definitions of probability. Terms such as *probability, chance,* or *likelihood* are commonplace, and most of us have a general notion of their meaning. A coin is tossed in the air, and we say that the chance of heads is 50/50. We roll a die and agree that we have 1 out of 6 chances of rolling a 4. In general, then, we can agree that probability reflects the likelihood of a particular outcome, with numbers close to 0 reflecting a very small chance of occurrence and numbers close to 1 indicating a very good chance of occurrence. But how do we define, and ultimately determine, probability?

Definitions of Probability

At least three formal definitions of probability can be identified:

Relative frequency definition. Probability can be defined in terms of relative frequency as the proportion of the time an event would occur over an infinite number of trials. In practical terms, the probability of an event can be estimated by using a large number of trials. As the number of trials increases, the relative frequency of occurrence approaches the actual probability of the event. Thus, the probability of rolling a 4 with a die can be estimated by observing the proportion of times that a 4 was rolled in a large number of trials (i.e., number of 4s/number of rolls). If the die were "fair," we would expect this relative frequency to approach 1/6 (0.166667) as the number of trials increases.

Deductive logic definition. The probability of an event can be determined logically from a consideration of the possible events and the total number of events. This can frequently be accomplished on the basis of symmetrical or geometric properties. For example, a coin has two symmetrical sides. Therefore, the probability of a head can be logically established as .5 by considering heads as one of two equivalent events.

Subjective definition. Probability can be defined subjectively in terms of an individual's certainty or degree of belief that an event will occur. For example, an individual may state that there is "only one chance in a hundred" that Notre Dame will beat Indiana in the NCAA basketball final. Thus, probability is established on the basis of an individual's knowledge or beliefs.

Definitions: discussion. The first two definitions of probability are objective. Different people using the same methods would arrive at the same conclusions about probability by using these definitions. In contrast, using a subjective definition, different people may arrive at quite different estimates of probability for a given event. As a consequence, subjective probabilities have limited application in statistics.

In comparing objective definitions of probability, the deductive logic definition does not provide a basis for verifying estimates of probability without relying on relative frequency. For example, we can establish the probability of heads when flipping a coin as .5 on the basis of its two symmetrical sides. How do we check to determine whether this estimate is accurate? We flip the coin a large number of times and determine what percentage of the time the coin flip resulted in heads. A further limitation of the deductive logic approach is that it is often difficult or impossible to apply this technique to complex events. For example, deductive logic provides little help in determining the probability that a patient with major depressive disorder has a comorbid anxiety disorder. As a consequence, most statistical applications rely on the relative frequency definition of probability.

Normal Distribution

The *normal distribution,* also referred to as a *Gaussian distribution,* provides the basis for many of the inferential statistics that are described later in this chapter. First, the characteristics of the normal distribution are highlighted. Second, the importance of the normal distribution to inferential statistics is considered.

The normal distribution is a theoretical distribution defined in terms of a mathematical function referred to as the *normal probability density function* (see, for example, Hays 1973). As such, the normal distribution is a continuous distribution that contains values ranging from negative infinity to positive infinity. The normal distribution curve is a bell-shaped, unimodal, symmetrical curve, suggesting that the mean, median, and mode all have the same value. A particularly useful characteristic of the normal distribution is that the percentage of observations within any given interval can be determined. A standard normal curve is shown in Figure 6–1.

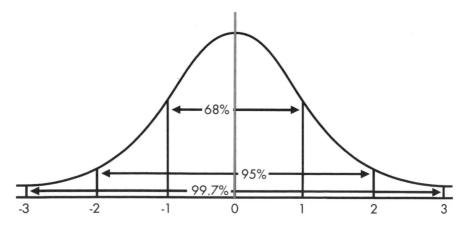

Figure 6–1.   Standard normal curve.

Approximately 68% of the observations fall within one standard deviation above and below the mean, approximately 95% of the observations fall within two standard deviations above and below the mean, and nearly 99% of all observations fall within three standard deviations above and below the mean. A table of standard normal distribution areas is provided in Table 6–1.

This table is referred to as a *standard* normal distribution because it references a normal distribution with a mean of 0 and a standard deviation of 1.0. By using this table, the proportion of observations within any given interval can be determined. For example, the area between 1.0 and 1.5 standard deviations can be determined by subtracting the area for $z = 1.0$ (.3413) from the area for $z = 1.5$ (.4332). The result (.0919) indicates that just over 9% of all observations fall between 1 and 1.5 standard deviations above the mean.

Importance of the Normal Distribution

The normal distribution is important for a number of reasons:

1. The first reason is that a number of naturally occurring distributions are approximately normally distributed. One example includes the distribution of certain human characteristics, such as height, weight, IQ, and serum cholesterol. These distributions are obviously not exactly normal; however, their relative frequencies have been shown to be very close to a normal distribution. A second example that closely resembles a normal distribution is the distribution of errors, such as errors of measurement or discrimination. For example, if a large number of subjects are asked to mark the midpoint of a horizontal line, and their responses are graphed in terms of a frequency distribution, the resultant distribution would be approximately normal. It should be pointed out that the normal distribution cannot be considered "nature's rule," since many naturally occurring distributions do not resemble a normal distribution.

2. The second reason is that normal distribution serves as a good approximation for a number of other theoretical distributions. These theoretical distributions are often extremely complicated and cumbersome. The normal distribution often provides a simple, time-saving method of approximation. One example is the binomial distribution, which is used to determine the likelihood of a given outcome over a series of successive independent trials. The normal distribution is frequently used to provide an approximation for the binomial distribution, significantly reducing the calculations required to perform the test.

Table 6–1. Standard normal distribution

z	.00	.01	.02	.03	.04	.05	.06	.07	.08	.09
0.0	.0000	.0040	.0080	.0120	.0160	.0199	.0239	.0279	.0319	.0359
0.1	.0398	.0438	.0478	.0517	.0557	.0596	.0636	.0675	.0714	.0753
0.2	.0793	.0832	.0871	.0910	.0948	.0987	.1026	.1064	.1103	.1141
0.3	.1179	.1217	.1255	.1293	.1331	.1368	.1406	.1443	.1480	.1517
0.4	.1554	.1591	.1628	.1664	.1700	.1736	.1772	.1808	.1844	.1879
0.5	.1915	.1950	.1985	.2019	.2054	.2088	.2123	.2157	.2190	.2224
0.6	.2257	.2291	.2324	.2357	.2389	.2422	.2454	.2486	.2517	.2549
0.7	.2580	.2611	.2642	.2673	.2704	.2734	.2764	.2794	.2823	.2852
0.8	.2881	.2910	.2939	.2967	.2995	.3023	.3051	.3078	.3106	.3133
0.9	.3159	.3186	.3212	.3238	.3264	.3289	.3315	.3340	.3365	.3389
1.0	.3413	.3438	.3461	.3485	.3508	.3531	.3554	.3577	.3599	.3621
1.1	.3643	.3665	.3686	.3708	.3729	.3749	.3770	.3790	.3810	.3820
1.2	.3849	.3869	.3888	.3907	.3925	.3944	.3962	.3980	.3997	.4015
1.3	.4032	.4049	.4066	.4082	.4099	.4115	.4131	.4147	.4162	.4177
1.4	.4192	.4207	.4222	.4236	.4251	.4265	.4279	.4292	.4306	.4319
1.5	.4332	.4345	.4357	.4370	.4382	.4394	.4406	.4418	.4429	.4441
1.6	.4452	.4463	.4474	.4484	.4495	.4505	.4515	.4525	.4535	.4545
1.7	.4554	.4564	.4573	.4582	.4591	.4599	.4608	.4616	.4625	.4633
1.8	.4641	.4649	.4656	.4664	.4671	.4678	.4686	.4693	.4699	.4706
1.9	.4713	.4719	.4726	.4732	.4738	.4744	.4750	.4756	.4761	.4767
2.0	.4772	.4778	.4783	.4788	.4793	.4798	.4803	.4808	.4812	.4817
2.1	.4821	.4826	.4830	.4834	.4838	.4842	.4846	.4850	.4854	.4857
2.2	.4861	.4864	.4868	.4871	.4875	.4878	.4881	.4884	.4887	.4890
2.3	.4893	.4896	.4898	.4901	.4904	.4906	.4909	.4911	.4913	.4916
2.4	.4918	.4920	.4922	.4925	.4927	.4929	.4931	.4932	.4934	.4936
2.5	.4938	.4940	.4941	.4943	.4945	.4946	.4948	.4949	.4951	.4952
2.6	.4953	.4955	.4956	.4957	.4959	.4960	.4961	.4962	.4963	.4964
2.7	.4965	.4966	.4967	.4968	.4969	.4970	.4971	.4972	.4973	.4974
2.8	.4974	.4975	.4976	.4977	.4977	.4978	.4979	.4979	.4980	.4981
2.9	.4981	.4982	.4982	.4983	.4984	.4984	.4985	.4985	.4986	.4986
3.0	.4987	.4987	.4987	.4988	.4988	.4989	.4989	.4989	.4990	.4990

3. The third reason has to do with sampling and a principle known as the *central limit theorem*. Consider a case in which a large number of samples of size N are drawn from the same finite population, the mean of each sample is calculated, and these means are used to form a new distribution of means, referred to as the *sampling distribution of means*. The central limit theorem states that, *regardless of the form of the original distribution, the distribution of means will be approximately normal when* N *is large*. This principle provides the foundation for interval estimation and a variety of inferential statistics, including *t* tests and analysis of variance.

4. The fourth reason has to do with its direct links to probability. Recall that the percentage of observations can be determined in a normal curve for any given interval. Also keep in mind that probability is defined in terms of the relative frequency of occurrence of an event over the long run. Given these considerations, what is the probability of randomly drawing an observation from a normal curve that is within 1 standard deviation above or below the mean? The answer is given in terms of the relative frequency of that event if we were to draw a random observation over a large number of trials. Since approximately 68% of all observations in a normal curve fall within this interval, the probability of that event is approximately .68.

Point Estimation

Point estimation is the use of a sample statistic to estimate the value of a population parameter. Recall that a sample statistic is a summary characteristic used to describe a sample, such as the sample mean or standard deviation. A population parameter is a summary characteristic used to describe a population. The basis of point estimation, therefore, is using a subset of the data to make inferences about some characteristic of the larger population.

What Makes a Good Estimator?

Four properties of a good estimator can be identified:

1. First, an estimator should be *unbiased*. A sample statistic is an unbiased estimator of a population parameter if, over a large number of samples, the mean of that sample statistic is equal to the value of the population parameter. In other words, over the long run, an unbiased estimator will average out to equal the population parameter.

2. A second property of a good estimator is *consistency*. A sample statistic is consistent if the probability of that statistic being close to the population parameter increases as the size of the sample increases. That is, the larger the sample, the more accurate the estimate.

3. A third property of a good estimator is *relative efficiency*. Relative efficiency provides a basis for comparing estimators. Suppose that two statistics are being considered as estimators for a population parameter. A large number of samples are drawn from that population. For each sample, the values for the two statistics are calculated. These values are used to create two new distributions, one for each statistic. These new distributions are referred to as *sampling distributions,* since they consist of observations obtained via sampling from a population. The more efficient statistic is the one for which the sampling distribution has a smaller standard deviation—or *standard error,* as it is called when used to describe a sampling distribution. The standard error is equal to the sample standard deviation divided by the square root of the sample size. Thus, relative efficiency expresses the tendency of a statistic to be closer to the population parameter—that is, more accurate over the long run in comparison with other statistics.

4. The final property of a good estimator is *sufficiency*. A sufficient estimator is one that cannot be improved by adding other aspects of the sample data.

Commonly Used Estimators

Sample mean. One of the most commonly used estimators in statistics is the *sample mean.* The sample mean is an unbiased estimator of the population mean: if a large number of samples is drawn from a population, the mean of the sampling distribution of means is equal to the population mean. The sample mean is also consistent: as the sample size increases, the standard error of the sampling distribution of means decreases. This can be shown by considering the formula for the standard error: the standard error is equal to the sample standard deviation divided by the square root of the sample size. As the sample size increases, the standard error becomes smaller. The mean is also efficient relative to other estimates of the population mean (e.g., median, mode), and it is sufficient in that it cannot be improved by adding other information about the sample.

Sample variance. In contrast to the sample mean, the *sample variance* is a biased estimator of the population variance, since, over the long run, the mean of the sampling distribution of variances is slightly lower than the population variance. An unbiased estimate of the population variance is obtained by dividing the sum of the squared deviations by $N-1$ instead of N. This corrected estimate meets all of the properties of a good estimator: unbiased, consistent, relatively efficient, and sufficient.

Interval Estimation

Point estimation provides us with a best guess at a population parameter. However, point estimation is limited in that it conveys no information about how accurate this estimate is likely to be. Consider an example: a researcher is interested in determining the average IQ of patients with Tourette's disorder in the United States. The researcher tests 40 patients with Tourette's disorder and finds that the mean IQ of these patients is 96 with a sample standard deviation of 15. Using point estimation, the researcher would conclude that 96 is the single best guess of the IQ for Tourette's disorder patients in the United States. However, a number of important questions remain unanswered: How accurate is this estimate? Is the mean IQ of patients with Tourette's disorder different from the mean IQ of the U.S. population in general? Point estimation provides us with a single best guess, but interval estimation can be used to answer questions like those posed here.

Confidence Intervals

Interval estimation is the specification of a range of values (i.e., an interval) based on a sample to make statements about our confidence that this interval contains the population parameter. These intervals are called *confidence intervals* (CIs). For example, we can determine the 95% CI for the previous example. The correct interpretation of this interval would be that if we were to draw repeated samples of 40 Tourette's disorder patients, 95% of those intervals would contain the population parameter—in this case, the mean IQ of all Tourette's disorder patients. Since we have only a single interval drawn from a single sample, we would be "95% confident" that our interval contained the mean IQ of all Tourette's disorder patients.

  To calculate a CI, we need three pieces of information:

1. Our "best guess" of the population parameter. We know that the mean of a sample is the single best guess as to the mean of the population. Thus, 96 is our single best guess as to the mean IQ of Tourette's disorder patients.

2. What the distribution of sample means would look like if we were to repeat the sampling process a large number of times.

   a. First, based on the central limit theorem, we know that this sampling distribution of means would be normally distributed, regardless of the distribution of the population.

   b. Next, from our knowledge of sampling distributions, we know that the standard error of the mean (i.e., the standard deviation of the sampling distribution of means) is equal to the population standard deviation divided by the square root of N (the sample size). Since the sample standard deviation is an unbiased estimate of the population standard deviation, in our previous example, the standard error of the mean (SEM) would be:

$$\text{SEM} = \frac{\text{sample standard deviation}}{\sqrt{N}} = \frac{15}{\sqrt{40}} = 2.37$$

3. The percent CI desired. Typical CIs are 95% and 99%.

These three pieces of information, along with our knowledge of the normal curve, can now be used to create a CI. We know that the sampling distribution would be normally distributed with a mean of 96 and a standard deviation of 2.37. Based on the standard normal distribution (Table 6–1), we know that 95% of the normal distribution falls within ±1.96 standard deviations of the mean (99% falls within ±2.58 standard deviations). Therefore,

95% CI = sample mean ± 1.96 (SEM) = 96 ± 1.96 (2.37) = 91.35 – 100.65

We are 95% confident that the IQ of all patients with Tourette's disorder falls within this range. We therefore cannot conclude that the IQ of Tourette's disorder patients is different from the IQ of the general population, since the interval contains the general population mean (i.e., 100).

One feature of the CI is that as the sample size increases, the CI becomes smaller. This is because the denominator of the SEM is the square root of the sample size (N). As N increases, the denominator likewise increases, reducing the SEM and narrowing the CI.

Hypothesis Testing

A third category of inferential statistics is *hypothesis testing*. It uses sample data to evaluate a statistical hypothesis about one or more population parameters.

Statistical hypotheses are precise statements about the population parameters.

For example, a statistical hypothesis about a *single population parameter* may be of the form:

Population mean = 78

or

Population variance > 100

Statistical hypotheses can also involve *more than one population parameter.* For example,

Population mean 1 > population mean 2

As a general rule, it is much easier to demonstrate that a hypothesis is false than to demonstrate that a hypothesis is true. Consider this simple hypothesis: All cows have four legs. To demonstrate that this hypothesis is true beyond any doubt, we would need to examine all cows. In contrast, to demonstrate that the hypothesis is false, we would only need to provide a single exception. It is this characteristic that provides the rationale for statistical hypothesis testing.

Research Hypotheses and Null Hypotheses

In hypothesis testing, our intent is typically to demonstrate that some relationship exists between variables, such as differences between groups or an association between variables. We can develop specific statistical hypotheses about these relationships, such as those presented above. These hypotheses are referred to as *research hypotheses,* since they express the intent of the research. However, as explained previously, it is extremely difficult, if not impossible, to demonstrate that these hypotheses are true. Therefore, in hypothesis testing, we develop a hypothesis contrary to the research hypotheses, with the intent of demonstrating that this contrary hypothesis is false. This contrary hypothesis is referred to as the *null hypothesis* (symbolized as H_0). In tests of differences, the null hypothesis typically takes the form of a statement that there are no differences. For example,

Null hypothesis:

Population mean 1 = population mean 2

Research hypothesis:

Population mean 1 > population mean 2 (directional)

or

Population mean 1 ≠ population mean 2 (nondirectional)

In tests of association, the null hypothesis typically takes the form of a statement that there is no association. For example,

Null hypothesis:
  Correlation (population 1 and population 2) = 0
Research hypothesis:
  Correlation (population 1 and population 2) > 0 (directional)
or
  Correlation (population 1 and population 2) ≠ 0 (nondirectional)

Evaluating the Null Hypothesis

In hypothesis testing, the null hypothesis is evaluated by specifying decision rules for rejecting or not rejecting the null hypothesis. Rejecting the null hypothesis involves concluding that the null hypothesis is false on the basis of the sample data. In contrast, not rejecting the null hypothesis means only that there is not sufficient information on the basis of the sample data to conclude that the null hypothesis is false; it is not equivalent to concluding that the null hypothesis is true.

Consider the following example: a researcher is comparing impulsiveness in bulimic patients and control subjects. The research samples 40 bulimic patients and 40 control subjects. The following hypotheses are developed:
  Null hypothesis:
    Mean impulsiveness (bulimic patients) = mean impulsiveness (control subjects)
  Research hypothesis:
    Mean impulsiveness (bulimic patients) > mean impulsiveness (control subjects)
Note that a directional research hypothesis is specified because the researcher expects the bulimic patients to score higher (rather than just differently) on impulsiveness, judging from previous research and theory.

The decision process can now be presented graphically in a 2×2 table, Table 6–2. The table represents the four possible results of hypothesis testing. Two of the four possible decisions are correct; two represent incorrect decisions.

Correctly rejecting the null hypothesis. If the mean impulsiveness score were higher in the population of bulimic patients than in the general population, the researcher could correctly reject the null hypothesis. In this case, on the basis of the sample data, the researcher would correctly conclude that impulsiveness is greater in bulimic patients than in control subjects.

The probability of correctly rejecting the null hypothesis is referred to as *statistical power*. Statistical power is a function of three variables: sample size, effect size, and α.

- First, statistical power increases as the sample size increases. The larger the sample, the greater is the proportion of the population that your sample represents, and the greater is the probability of identifying a "real" relationship between variables or differences between groups.
- The second factor influencing statistical power is effect size, which refers to the strength of the actual relationship in the population(s): the size of the difference between groups or the strength of the association between variables. The greater the effect size, the greater is the ability to identify that relationship on the basis of the sample data.
- The third factor that influences statistical power is α. Statistical power is inversely related to α. In considering α, we must turn to the second of the four cells in Table 6–2.

Incorrectly rejecting the null hypothesis: Type I error. A second possible outcome is incorrectly rejecting the null hypothesis. This is referred to as a *Type I error,* which is a false positive error–that is, an incorrect conclusion that a relationship exists. In the example above, the researcher would conclude on the basis of the sample data that impulsiveness is greater in bulimic patients, when in fact there are no differences in impulsiveness between bulimic patients and general populations. Decision rules are typically constructed in such a way that the probability of a Type I error, referred to as α, does not exceed .05 or .01. The construction of decision rules is considered further below.

Correctly not rejecting the null hypothesis. A third possible outcome of hypothesis testing is correctly not rejecting the null hypothesis. In our example, on the basis of the sample data, the researcher would decide that there is not sufficient evidence to conclude that the population of bulimic patients differs in impulsiveness from the general population. The probability of making this decision, given that the null hypothesis is in fact true, is $1 - \alpha$.

Table 6–2.   Hypothesis testing

Decision	True state of affairs	
	H_0 true	H_0 false
Reject H_0	Type I error $(p = \alpha)$	Correct $(p = 1 - \beta = \text{power})$
Not reject H_0	Correct $(p = 1 - \alpha)$	Type II error $(p = \beta)$

Note. p = probability.

Incorrectly not rejecting the null hypothesis: Type II error. The fourth possible outcome of hypothesis testing is incorrectly not rejecting the null hypothesis. In this case, the researcher would conclude on the basis of the sample data that there is not sufficient evidence to suggest a difference in impulsiveness between the population of bulimic patients and the general population, whereas in fact this difference does exist. This type of error is referred to as a *Type II error,* which is a false-negative error. The probability of a Type II error (referred to as β), given that the null hypothesis is false, is 1 − statistical power.

Statistical Significance

We now turn to the issue of statistical significance. What does it mean when it is stated that a statistical test "is significant?" How do we determine what is and what is not statistically significant? To answer these questions, we must consider a six-step process that is the basis of all hypothesis testing. These six steps will be considered in relation to our research example.

Step 1: Specify the null hypothesis and the research hypothesis. In the example discussed previously, the hypotheses are as follows:

 Mean impulsiveness (bulimic patients) = mean impulsiveness (control subjects)

 or

 Mean impulsiveness (bulimic patients) − mean impulsiveness (control subjects) = 0

 Research hypothesis:

 Mean impulsiveness (bulimic patients) > mean impulsiveness (control subjects)

Note that the two forms of the null hypothesis above are equivalent. Also, keep in mind that these hypotheses refer to population parameters, not to sample statistics.

Step 2: Assume that the null hypothesis is true.

 This point seems simple, but it is extremely important. Statistical significance can only be determined by assuming that the null hypothesis is true.

Step 3: Determine what the distribution would be if the sampling process were repeated over a large number of trials.

 In the example, the researcher sampled 40 bulimic patients and 40 control subjects. Suppose that the researcher subtracts the control sample mean impulsiveness score from the bulimic sample mean impulsiveness score, then places that difference in a new distribution. Suppose further that this same sampling process is repeated over a large number of trials. For each trial, the difference in mean impulsiveness between the samples is placed in the new distribution. What would this new distribution look like?

First, from the central limit theorem, we know that the distribution would be approximately normal. Next, because we are assuming that the null hypothesis is true (i.e., Step 2), we know that the mean of this new distribution would be 0 (from the null hypothesis in Step 1). Finally, from sampling distribution theory, we know that the standard deviation of this distribution (i.e., the SEM) can be estimated by the following equation:

$$ \text{SEM} = \sqrt{\left(\text{sample SD}_{\text{bulimic}}{}^2 / N_{\text{bulimic}} \right) + \left(\text{sample SD}_{\text{control}}{}^2 / N_{\text{control}} \right)} $$

If the sample standard deviation for the bulimic sample is 10, and the sample standard deviation from the control sample is 8, then

$$ \text{SEM} = \sqrt{\left(\tfrac{10^2}{40} \right) + \left(\tfrac{8^2}{40} \right)} = 2.02 $$

Step 4: Choose an α level.

Recall that α is the probability of making a Type I error. Since we want to minimize the chances of making a false-positive error (i.e., mistakenly concluding that an effect is present), α levels are typically set at .05 or .01. We will use .01 for the current example.

Step 5: Determine decision rules for rejecting and not rejecting the null hypothesis.

Our decision rules must be such that, if the null hypothesis is true, the chance of making a Type I error is .01. We know that the sampling distribution of means for this example is normal, has a mean of 0, and has a standard error of 2.02. Keep in mind that a difference greater than 0 indicates that the mean impulsiveness score for the sample of bulimic patients is greater than the mean impulsiveness score for the control sample. Since the research hypothesis is that impulsiveness is greater in bulimic patients (i.e., a directional hypothesis), we want to choose a difference between samples such that, if the null hypothesis is true, a value this large would occur only about 1% of the time. In the standard normal table (Table 6–1), we see that a z-score of 2.33 is the point in the normal curve that demarcates the upper 1% of the distribution. That is, in a normal distribution, only 1% of the observations fall at or above 2.33 standard deviations above the mean. To translate this into a decision rule, multiply the SEM in the current example (2.02) by this value:

$$\text{Cut point} = 2.02 \ (2.33) = 4.71$$

The decision rules can now be specified. If the mean impulsiveness score for the bulimic patients is 4.71 points or more above the mean for control subjects, the null hypothesis is rejected; otherwise, the null hypothesis is not rejected.

Step 6: Make a decision based on the sample data.

We now can compare the mean impulsiveness scores for bulimic patients and control subjects. In the present example, the mean impulsiveness score for bulimic patients is 25.1 and that for control subjects is 19.6. The difference is 5.5. Since our difference (5.5) is larger than the cut point (4.71), we reject the null hypothesis and conclude that the mean impulsiveness score for bulimic patients is higher than for the general population.

We now can consider the question posed at the beginning of this discussion: the meaning of statistical significance. In the research example, statistical significance has the following interpretation:

Assuming that the null hypothesis is true, a difference of 5.5 or more points in mean impulsiveness scores between bulimic patients and control subjects will occur only 1% of the time.

Concluding Comments

Several important comments about hypothesis testing must now be made.

First, it is important to understand that all hypothesis testing follows this same process, implicitly if not explicitly. In practice, we often do not explicitly state the null hypothesis but merely assume a null hypothesis of no difference or no association. Likewise, we do not methodically determine the decision rules, but rather let the computer do the work. At the same time, however, each step in the process, whether explicitly stated or implicitly understood, is a necessary step in hypothesis testing.

A second point concerns step 3, the determination of the sampling distribution based on the null hypothesis. Different types of hypothesis testing require different methods of determining this distribution. It is beyond the scope of this book to consider these techniques. Interested readers are referred to Hays (1973) or Woolson (1987). Frankly, most readers of this book will not be interested in pursuing this topic in any detail, nor should they feel compelled to in order to have a basic understanding of hypothesis testing.

Table 6–3. Tests of differences

Dependent variable	1 group	Independent variable 2 groups Independent groups	Independent variable 2 groups Matched groups	Independent variable k groups Independent groups	Independent variable k groups Matched groups
Nominal	Binomial test χ^2 one-sample test	χ^2 test for 2 independent groups Fisher's exact test	McNemar test	χ^2 test for k independent groups	Cochran's Q test
Ordinal	One-sample runs test	Mann-Whitney U test Median test Wald-Wolfowitz runs test	Wilcoxon test Sign test	Kruskal-Wallis test	Friedman test
Interval/ratio	One-sample t test	Independent samples t test	Paired t test	One-way ANOVA	Repeated-measures ANOVA

Note. ANOVA = analysis of variance.

Tables 6–3 through 6–5 summarize some of the most frequently used statistical tests. Readers are encouraged to read more about these tests and the assumptions upon which they are based in Hays (1973), Seigel (1956), or Woolson (1987).

Table 6–3 presents commonly used tests of differences. Tests are organized in terms of the scale of measurement for the dependent and independent variables. A distinction is made within independent variables between independent and matched groups. Independent groups have no inherent connection between group members. In contrast, matched groups are characterized by some link or connection between group members. Examples of matched groups would be 1) husbands and wives and 2) probands and first-degree relatives.

Tests of association are used to describe relationships between variables; *tests of agreement* measure the extent of concordance between variables. Tests of agreement are frequently used to express reliability (e.g., interrater reliability).

Table 6–4 presents common tests of association and tests of agreement between two variables.

Table 6–4. Tests of association and tests of agreement for two variables

	Nominal	Ordinal	Interval/ratio
Nominal	Phi coefficient Contingency coefficient Cramer's V κ (kappa)		
Ordinal	⟵———	Spearman's rank order correlation	
	⟵———	Kendall's τ (tau)	
Interval/ratio	Point biserial correlation η (eta) *Intraclass correlation coefficient*		Pearson's r Simple regression

Note. Tests in roman type are tests of association; those in italic type are tests of agreement. Arrows indicate tests that are intended primarily for a specific variable (e.g., two nominal variables) but are also suitable for another combination.

Table 6–5. Measures of association: multiple independent variables

Dependent variable	Independent variables		
	Nominal	**Ordinal**	**Interval/ratio**
Nominal	Logistic regression (2 dependent variable categories)		
	Discriminant function analysis (k dependent variable categories)		
Ordinal	Probit regression		
Interval/ratio	Multiple linear regression		

Table 6–5 presents tests of association for a single dependent variable and multiple independent variables.

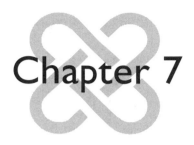

Chapter 7

Research Support

Introduction: Overview of NIH

In excess of 90% of non-industry-sponsored biomedical research in the United States is funded by the federal government, through various mechanisms. The usual source of funding for clinical researchers in psychiatry is three institutes that are part of the National Institutes of Health: the National Institute of Mental Health, the National Institute of Drug Abuse, and the National Institute on Alcohol Abuse and Alcoholism.

The federal bureaucracy is notoriously complex; therefore, a reasonable place to start is an overview of the various agencies involved and how they relate to one another (Figure 7–1).

The National Institutes of Health (NIH), which accounts for much of the extramural research funding, is one of the administrative agencies in DHHS. *Extramural* funds go to investigators outside NIH; *intramural* funds are spent for in-house research, primarily at the NIH campus in Bethesda, Maryland. Under NIH, there are a total of 24 institutes (Table 7–1).

Until the last few years, the three institutes primarily affiliated with mental health and substance abuse issues (NIMH, NIAAA, and NIDA) were separated from NIH and placed in the Alcohol, Drug Abuse, and Mental Health Administration (ADAMHA). These three institutes have now been incorporated into NIH proper.

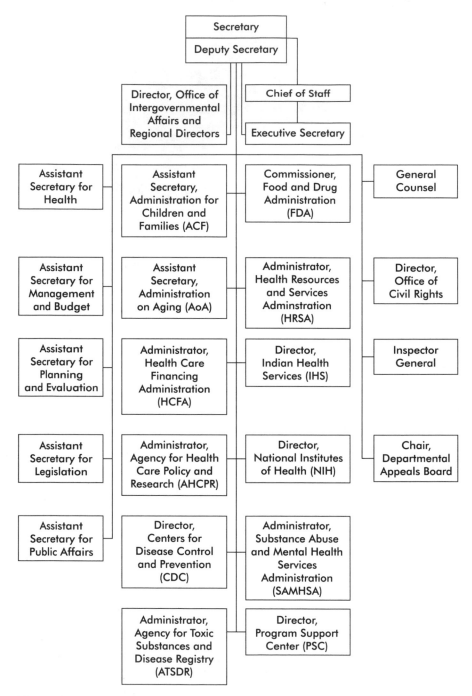

Figure 7–1. Organization chart of the Department of Health and Human Services.

Table 7–1. NIH institutes and other divisions

1. National Cancer Institute (NCI)
2. National Heart, Lung, and Blood Institute (NHLBI)
3. National Institute of Allergy and Infectious Disease (NIAID)
4. National Institute of General Medical Services (NIGMS)
5. National Institute of Diabetes and Digestive and Kidney Diseases (NIDDK)
6. National Institute of Neurological Disorders and Stroke (NINDS)
7. National Institute of Mental Health (NIMH)
8. National Institute of Child Health and Development (NICHD)
9. National Institute of Drug Abuse (NIDA)
10. National Institute on Aging (NIA)
11. National Institute of Dental Research (NIDR)
12. National Human Genome Research Institute (NHGRI)
13. National Eye Institute (NEI)
14. National Institute on Deafness and Other Communication Disorders (NIDCD)
15. The Fogarty International Center
16. National Institute of Environmental Health and Sciences (NIEHS)
17. National Library of Medicine (NLM)
18. Division of Computer Research and Technology
19. National Institute of Arthritis and Musculoskeletal and Skin Diseases (NIAMS)
20. National Institute of Nursing Research (NINR)
21. Division of Research Grants
22. National Institute on Alcohol Abuse and Alcoholism (NIAAA)
23. The Warren Grant Magnuson Clinical Center
24. National Center for Research Resources (NCRR)

Process of Grant Application Submission

Most psychiatry departments have copies of the materials that are required as part of a grant submission. (For details on where and how to request grant packets, see Appendix F.)

When an application is received in Washington, D.C. (original plus 5 copies), it is first sorted by topic and assigned to an institute, then within the institute to an Initial Review Group (Figure 7–2).

The title of a grant application may be very important in this regard. The application is assigned to an executive secretary for that committee and is scheduled for the next committee review meeting. All grant applications assigned for review are sent to all the committee members in advance of the meeting. However, most of the grant applications are read only superficially by most committee members, except the grant applications to which reviewers are assigned as first, second, or third reviewers. These individuals read these assigned grant applications very carefully and also read all the appendix material. They are responsible for leading the discussion of these grant applications at the time of the committee meeting. If there is not sufficient expertise on the committee to review an application, additional ad hoc reviewers may be assigned. Their reviews may be mailed to the committee, or if their input is thought to be particularly important, they may join the committee by conference call or may be invited to actually attend the committee meeting. In unusual circumstances, grant applications may be assigned to special review committees.

The applications are reviewed by the committee for scientific and technical merit and are assigned a rating. As of this writing, the system dictates that the committee assign the application a number from 1.0 to 5.0, 1.0 being a perfect score, and that each member vote individually in writing. In the last few years, a streamlined system has been adopted: applications that would be scored 3.0 or greater (meaning they are thought to be less competitive) have been so designated early in the meeting, and they are discussed only briefly at the meeting unless a member asks for a complete review. It was hoped that approximately half the applications would fall into this group and that the committee's deliberations would then focus on the competitive applications.

On the basis of the written evaluations brought to the committee, the discussion by the reviewers and other committee members, and any additional material that develops during the course of the discussion, "pink sheets" (they are no longer pink) are subsequently written by the executive secretary of the committee, usually incorporating reviewers' comments verbatim. The

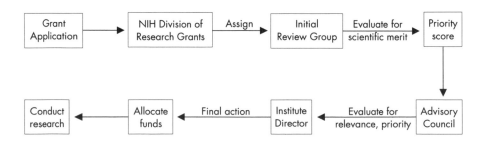

Figure 7–2. Review process for grant applications.

applications that are approved and that receive low percentile rankings are then reviewed by an advisory council for program balance and priority relative to issues of funding. Occasionally these committees will fund out of order, taking into account an institute's special missions, but generally this procedure accounts for 10% or less of the applications. In general, the grant applications with the lowest scores (closest to 1.0) are funded.

 Grant applications not approved can be resubmitted only two times, for a total of three submissions.

Writing Grant Applications

The section provides a brief introduction to the preparation of grant applications for external funding. It specifically addresses the preparation of applications for grants under R01, the primary grant mechanism of the National Institute of Health. These are single-center research grants that account for most of the grant applications reviewed and funded. Because of the fact that some of this section is less relevant to other types of submissions, details regarding other grant mechanisms should be examined as well on the NIH Web site (www.nih.gov). Before turning to specific parts of grant applications, we'll first list some general rules that may be useful.

Rule 1: Be Thick-Skinned

The process of preparing, submitting, having reviewed, and obtaining feedback on a grant application can be an intimidating and, at times, humiliating experience. As with many other things in academic medicine (and life in general), experience counts, and the first experience of many beginning investigators is not uncommonly to be at least disappointed, and at times hurt, by comments they receive about their proposals. It is far better to go into the process knowing that when first submitting an application, you will receive a great deal of feedback, often much of it negative. Bear in mind that even well-established, productive researchers with strong grant histories have trouble getting funding. This makes the task of obtaining funding particularly daunting for the younger investigators. However, since obtaining funding frequently ends up being a long-term process, it is probably best to start as early as possible, knowing that one's proposals will usually need to be significantly modified, polished, and resubmitted once or twice before being funded.

Rule 2: Keep the Scope of the Project Focused

Grand, elegant, creative schemes are fun in fantasy, but generally don't translate into good grants. An ordered, systematic protocol designed to answer one specific question, or at most a few specific questions, is much more likely to find favor, because it is much more likely to be completed and to yield significant results. Keep it simple.

Rule 3: Use All The Space You Can

On an RO1 request, there are certain page limitations, which have varied somewhat in the last few years. Most investigators feel constrained, for example, by the limitation on the methodology and design section to a certain suggested number of pages, and these investigators have difficulty cutting their grant applications down to fit the limits. On the other hand, when a grant proposal uses fewer pages than allotted, reviewers may logically assume that the investigator has not reviewed all the necessary literature, has not included all the necessary details of the experiment, or has not adequately described the data analysis techniques. A good rule of thumb is that if you include everything you need to include, you won't have enough room. Therefore, if you find you're not filling the allotted space, chances are there are things you are not thinking about. Get help.

Rule 4: Sell Your Idea

Scientists at times pull back from the idea of salesmanship. What we are suggesting by *salesmanship* is not selling snake oil, but selling a good idea and the resultant good proposal. You should be enthusiastic about your ideas and feel that they are important and that your work will both offer significant contributions to the field and develop into an ongoing program of research for you. You need to convince the reviewers about these points as well, so that they will understand your ideas, share your enthusiasm, believe that this area of inquiry will not be a dead end, and conclude that the result will contribute significantly to the field. Emphasize not only what you intend to do but why you are not doing other things. Putting together a grant protocol involves choices—choosing populations, choosing instruments, choosing outcome measures—and it is important not only to defend the choices you've made but at times also to indicate why other choices were ruled out. For example, why are certain patient populations to be excluded? Why aren't you using other instruments? Why have certain data analysis approaches been chosen?

Rule 5: Repeat and Emphasize

It is often useful to reiterate certain key ideas and concepts when writing a proposal and to place emphasis several times on certain central ideas, by repetition or other means (headings, italic type, bold type).

Rule 6: Be Clear

A grant submission is not the place to elaborate circuitous or oblique theoretical constructs. Submissions should be clear, concise, and practical, and the ideas put forth in the application should flow logically and build throughout the proposal.

Rule 7: Get Input

It is important for beginning investigators to have experienced grant application writers review their proposal (as many individuals as possible, as many times as possible). It is also often useful to have experienced grant application writers who don't work in your area as readers of the application, since their reading provides a good test of the clarity of the ideas. If a sophisticated researcher can't grasp the concepts, the proposal needs serious revision. However, it is also obviously useful to have those with a great deal of experience in the area of focus review the grant application and offer their criticisms and ideas.

Elements in a Grant Proposal

We now turn to specific elements in a proposal that must be considered in preparing it.

Title

The title should be brief, specific, and—most important—not misleading. Remember that the title of the proposal may determine to which study section it will be assigned for review. This may prove crucial in determining whether the proposal is reviewed by those best able to review it properly.

Abstract

The abstract should succinctly summarize the entire proposal, including aims, significance, experimental design, and expected outcome. Some granting agencies will have the primary reviewer read the abstract aloud so that other reviewers who may not have read the application in its entirety will hear a brief description. Therefore, read the abstract aloud. How does it sound? Does it adequately describe what you plan to do and why?

Specific Aims

First describe what the research is intended to accomplish: What is the scientific problem that is addressed by the research? It is important to specifically articulate hypotheses (again, they should be limited in number). Then address the significance of the research: How does this study fit into the big picture? Why is the proposed methodology particularly important? How well do the proposed experiments fill gaps in knowledge of the subject, and why is it important to fill these gaps? How can this area of study be pursued further in programmatic research, regardless of the specific outcome here?

Three or four specific aims is certainly a reasonable number, but ten or more may engender the response that the proposal is too ambitious or diffuse. Grant protocols are rarely criticized for being too focused or limited in approach, but they are often criticized for being too diffuse and for not having well-developed hypotheses.

Background and Significance

First it is important to know that the literature review is complete (or at least representative) and current. Those reviewing the proposal will often be among those active in this field of research, and they will usually know the most recently published results (and often the most recent unpublished results as well). Therefore, one needs to demonstrate a rigorous and broad-based understanding of the literature, how it fits together, its limitations and strengths, and how the proposed work will fill gaps in the current knowledge base. In keeping with the notion that experts in the field may be reviewing the work, consideration can be given to obtaining a list of current NIH committee membership. If you have a good idea which committee may receive the proposal, you may be able to figure out who one or more of the primary reviewers are likely to be. It is obviously in your best interest to make sure that any work they have done in the area is appropriately cited.

It is much easier for reviewers to find references in the text rather than having them numbered and having to search at the end of the proposal. Also, some investigators find it useful to divide the background and significance section into subsections with specific subtitles.

Some beginning investigators make the mistake of attempting to prove the worth of their own ideas by being overly critical of the works of others in the field. This is particularly true when criticisms are made of work that may have been done 5 or 10 years before, when standards in the field had not progressed to the current level. It is important to remember that all our research is based on the work of others, and therefore being fair and not overly critical regarding the work of others is appropriate. It is also politically astute, given the possible reviewers of proposals and manuscripts.

In this section it is important to highlight your work and the work of the other investigators named in the proposal, as well as contributions from researchers other than the investigators named in your proposal who work in your institution in related areas. This feature of your proposal will demonstrate a broad-based interest in the area in your facility or department.

Preliminary Data/Progress Reports

If the grant is a renewal, demonstrated progress on the previous grant is obviously of extreme importance, including not only publications but manuscripts, presentations, and other unpublished work completed before resubmission. In particular, if unexpected problems arose that resulted in changes in the original experimental design, these should be highlighted and defended in order to justify the current approach. It is important to demonstrate that timely progress is being made relative to the amount of time asked for in the previous funded proposal and that the work is proceeding in a logical manner.

Even for new applications, preliminary data are highly desirable, if not a necessity. Any preliminary data sets related to the proposal should be included. What one is attempting here is to prove to the committee not only that the current project is feasible but that the investigator is an active researcher who has worked in related areas and can do the sort of work called for in the proposal.

Often, program officers allow you to provide updates of data after the submission of the proposal but before the committee meeting. If you are permitted to do this, it is highly desirable to send in more information. This allows you to update the application, demonstrates your continued interest in the project and continued activity in the area, and underscores your continued desire and need for further funding.

In summary, the preliminary data section should be written in a way that will convince the committee that the investigator is capable of doing the studies, is interested in the area, and can do the work.

Experimental Design and Methods

Generally it is useful to separate methods of assessment from experimental design. It is also important to remember that flowcharts, figures, and tables are extremely helpful in summarizing complex design issues for reviewers.

The design sections can be broken up into various components, which are used as titles. For example, the following few sections are headed by the type of titles that might be included in a proposal, and the text discusses the content of such sections.

1. Methods

a. Sample populations and controls

It is important to demonstrate that the proposed sample population is appropriate for the protocol, that the sampling techniques are acceptable, and that there is an adequate comparison or control group. It is also important to document the availability of subjects and the feasibility of obtaining the proposed sample size. For example, couples with *folie à deux* may offer several interesting possibilities for research, but the likelihood of accumulating a significant number of such couples in a reasonable period of time is very low. The availability of subject samples leads many clinical investigators to superimpose the structure of their ongoing research programs on specialized clinical populations, such as those in anxiety disorder clinics, eating disorder programs, or mood disorder clinics.

The estimate of sample size is extremely important, and power analyses are now expected in clinical protocols. This estimate is a statistical technique whereby one can calculate the necessary sample size for answering questions, given certain other variables(e.g., effect size).

It is also important to carefully stipulate the inclusion and exclusion criteria and why they were chosen. This topic should address the presence or absence of certain comorbid conditions (e.g.: Can individuals be included in a protocol for major depressive disorders if they have had manic episodes and also meet criteria for bipolar disorder? How about subjects with borderline personality disorder?). The topic should also include age (e.g., do you intend to use adolescents, a group that will require attention to issues involving informed consent?). Do you want to stratify the sample on certain variables such as age, gender, or socioeconomic status? If so, sample sizes and power analyses need to be completed on the individual cells that result from such stratification.

The current standard is to include both men and women and both children and adults in clinical studies unless the exclusion of gender or age groups can be justified.

b. Measurement

It is highly important to make sure that measures are appropriate for the sample being studied and to include evidence of adequate psychometric properties for instruments (e.g., validity, reliability). Why were other instruments not used (particularly if they are commonly used in this field of research)? Keep in mind also that it is almost always better to use an extant instrument, even if it is not perfect, than to develop an instrument without existing validity or reliability data. It is also important to remember that structured clinical interviews for psychiatric diagnosis are now expected. If there is something you want to do, such as obtaining data on a new questionnaire that you have designed that does not significantly increase any risks to subjects but that you would have difficulty defending in a grant application, don't put it in the proposal, but reconsider it as an add-on to the project later, although its use will still require Institutional Review Board (IRB) approval (see Chapter 8).

c. Data collection

It is important to be sure that patient flow will be adequate for completing the protocol in the time proposed in the grant application. A small chart or table documenting intended patient flow can prove quite useful.

2. Study design

It is important to ensure that the design to be followed in the study is appropriate to the questions being asked—that it will answer the hypotheses that were put forth at the beginning of the application. If the methodology is standard, it can be dealt with somewhat superficially, but if it is novel, it must be described in sufficient detail to demonstrate that it has been adequately grounded in prior experience and shown to be successful. Preliminary data are particularly important here. Investigators must defend their choices and in particular attempt to anticipate potential problems and how they would be dealt with. It is highly important here to think as a reviewer: What could possibly go wrong? How would the investigator deal with it? It is very reassuring for reviewers, when they are reading an application and questions come to mind, to have those questions answered in the proposal.

Data Analysis

The data analysis approach needs to be outlined in detail and well referenced. It must be clear enough to be understandable to all members of the committees, yet sophisticated enough to satisfy the members who are particularly interested in data analysis techniques. How will the data be obtained? Where will the data be stored? How will the quality of the data be checked? How will each specific hypothesis be tested? In addition, carefully differentiate primary from secondary or post-hoc analyses.

Human Subjects

The population to be studied and its characteristics should be described in detail, including number, source, age, sex, ethnicity, and general health status. Inclusion criteria should be reviewed, and the use of any special or high-risk populations should be documented (e.g., institutionalized subjects, those with mental retardation). Rules regarding the use of men, women, children, and minorities in research have been in a state of flux, and it is important to be aware of the most recent requirements in this regard. As mentioned, the current standard is to include both genders and both children and adults, unless the exclusion of an age group or gender can be justified. It is also a current standard to have a specific plan for minority recruitment for most studies.

It is necessary to discuss in detail the nature and likelihood of potential risks, regardless of type. This would include physical risk, such as that from medications; psychological risks, such as the use of techniques that would induce stress or the use of instruments which might ask upsetting questions; legal risks, if potentially compromising data are to be obtained; and any other risks to which the subject might be exposed.

Procedures to protect the rights and welfare of subjects—including obtaining consent, maintaining confidentiality, and other procedures such as screening and debriefing of subjects—should be reviewed.

Review committees can express *comments* on human subject issues if they feel the problem is not unduly serious; these comments will be communicated in the pink sheets, to be corrected by the investigator. *Concerns,* however, require the program staff not to fund the research until the issues are addressed.

In all human subject considerations, risks versus benefits must be carefully weighed.

Resources and Environment

It is important to document that the equipment and facilities are currently available to carry out the protocol and will remain so for the duration of the project. It is also important to document that the investigator will have access to consultation and guidance from other investigators, particularly if the investigator is junior and relatively inexperienced. The rule is to include rather than exclude clinical resources, computer facilities, office space, equipment and supplies, and anything else that could be of relevance.

Budget

For grant applications that do not exceed $250,000 direct costs in any one year, the budget section has been simplified, and few details have to be provided with the application.

With larger grants, the most common budget problem is the lack of justification. It is important for the investigator to carefully document the need for each budgetary item. Composite figures should not be given; instead, the actual calculations should be shown. For example, if a half-time Ph.D. position is requested for administration of semistructured interviews, it is important to document that 50% of an individual's time for 1 year is actually necessary, given the number of interviews, the time it takes to administer the interview, and so forth. Areas that will draw particular attention are foreign travel, which is often not justified; costly supplies and equipment, which may already be present on site; and large amounts for consultant costs, although appropriate amounts for consultation may prove very helpful to an applicant.

Many proposals are quite expensive, but the issue that usually concerns the committee is not the cost but the justification for the cost. Spend the time when preparing the protocol to make sure that you have accounted for everything you need and have justified it. This will save much heartache later if, in one case, the requested budget is cut in the actual grant because of inadequate justification, or, in another case, if the proposal is funded and you discover later that you have asked for too little money.

Relative to duration of funding, most proposals that ask for longer than a 3-year time commitment need to be carefully justified by the research design, although funding up to 5 years is possible. Again, the use of a figure with timelines can be very helpful in this area of the proposal.

Appendix

The appendix should be well thought out and should include everything that is of direct relevance to the protocol, including copies of all measures, detailed treatment manuals in projects that involve treatments, further details on issues for which there is not adequate space in the application proper, and evidence of scientific productivity, including reprints and manuscripts. Only the primary reviewers receive the appendix material, but they review it with care, and the appendix can supply the additional detail lacking in the proposal, which can be very convincing to a reviewer.

Conclusions

Seeking and obtaining research support for one's research is usually the most daunting task facing a beginning investigator. The forms are intimidating, the system is confusing, and the comments from colleagues can at times be discouraging. However, people manage to obtain support; and in some ways the task may be becoming easier—particularly with the growing emphasis on providing opportunities for more junior investigators.

Dive in, get advice, familiarize yourself with the forms, and don't hesitate to call NIH (see Appendix F for contact information). People there are usually informative, supportive, and very approachable.

CHAPTER 8

Use of Human Subjects in Research: The Institutional Review Board

Introduction

On first encountering the Institutional Review Board (IRB), the investigator new to the process of research involving human subjects often regards this entity merely as another impediment to getting the research project started (requiring yet another complex form to fill out) and at times also as some sinister extension of the federal bureaucracy. The former is in practical terms true: the necessity of involving the IRB often does slow things down, and the form at first can take a great deal of time. However, IRBs are far from sinister, and the beginning investigator will have taken a great step forward in a research career if he or she pauses early on to consider the importance of the IRB—in protecting human subjects, in protecting researchers, and in helping to maintain high standards in research. By reviewing the history of the protection of human subjects in research and the events that led to the current regulations in this area, we hope to demystify the IRB and provide some perspective on its mandate as it relates to investigators and their research subjects.

Later in this chapter we review current federal regulations governing the IRB and their effect on the investigator. The specifics of the informed consent are reviewed, along with the precautions that must be taken in working with vulnerable populations. These sections should further clarify the nature of the interaction between the investigator and the IRB, simplifying the process of seeking and receiving IRB approval and also suggesting the position that IRBs are a necessary, important, and often helpful part of the process of research.

The Emergence of Ethical Codes Concerning Research on Human Subjects

The Nuremberg Code (see Appendix A) is generally regarded as the document that marked the beginning of formal and systematic thinking concerning the protection of human subjects in research during the modern era. This document came about during the course of the doctors' trial (December 1946–August 1947) initiated by the postwar Nuremberg military tribunal (Annas and Grodin 1992). This trial, the so-called medical case, was one of many (and not to be confused with the more famous trial involving military officers of the Third Reich) that took place in postwar Germany. The prosecution's primary charge against the 23 defendants was that they had engaged in unethical research in using nonconsenting prisoners. The practical problem was that a generally acknowledged code of ethics by which to judge the defendants did not exist at the time of the trial. In answer to this deficiency the experts for the prosecution, Drs. Leo Alexander and Andrew Ivy, offered before the trial's closing arguments what became known as the Nuremberg Code. Apparently, to lend the document credibility, Dr. Ivy, who was associated with the American Medical Association, arranged for a truncated version of the Code to be published in the Journal of the American Medical Association early in the course of the trial (Annas and Grodin 1992). The Nuremberg Code (see Appendix A) called for informed consent, voluntary participation by subjects, and the ability to withdraw from an experiment at any time. These elements formed the basis for subsequent work in the area of codifying the ethics of research.

Despite the vivid descriptions of the atrocities committed by the Nazis that emerged during the doctors' trial, neither the trial nor the Nuremberg Code received much attention in the American press during the trial or in the 15 years that followed. However, as we will see, it was common then to conduct research projects that by today's standards would be unethical.

In the postwar period, interest in ethical behavior for physicians emerged independent of the Nuremberg trials. In 1947 the World Medical Association (WMA) was founded and soon concerned itself with developing professional ethical codes and guidelines. Following some initial articles addressing the professional behavior of physicians, such as "The Dedication of the Physician" in 1948 (Annas and Grodin 1992, p. 154), the WMA developed professional guidelines for experimentation on human beings, culminating in the Declaration of Helsinki in June 1964 (see Appendix B), which was formally adopted in the 18th Assembly of the WMA. The Declaration of Helsinki is said to have been greatly influenced by the Nuremberg Code (Levine 1991) but goes beyond it in a number of ways: primarily, it differentiates between research with potential therapeutic value and research for the advancement of scientific knowledge, suggesting that the same ethical principles must be followed when combining experimentation with therapeutic care as must be adhered to when experimenting with healthy volunteers (Annas and Grodin 1992).

The Belmont Report

Although the Nuremberg Code and the Declaration of Helsinki provided valuable guidance in our thinking about the ethical treatment of research subjects, on a practical basis they had no legally binding authority. While physicians grappled with these difficult ethical concerns, the federal government moved in parallel to codify these ideas into regulations. As is covered later in this chapter, a number of events during the 1960s and 1970s galvanized the U.S. government's interest in the treatment of research subjects. One result of this interest was passage by Congress of the National Research Act, which in July 1974 established the National Commission for the Protection of Human Subjects of Biomedical and Behavioral Research (from here on in this chapter called the Commission). In the wake of *Roe v. Wade* in 1972, the Commission had the specific charge of studying the nature of research conducted with fetuses, but it was also given the more general mandate of identifying "the basic ethical principles which should underlie the conduct of biomedical and behavioral research involving human subjects"(Annas and Grodin 1992, p. 187). The Commission met from 1975 through 1978 (to be replaced by the President's Commission, 1980–1983) and produced a series of reports and recommendations submitted to the secretary of the Department of Health, Education and Welfare (DHEW). The recommendations were intended to form the basis for developing new regulations to be promulgated by DHEW (which in 1979 was divided into the Department of Health and Human Services [DHHS] and the Department of Education). Although DHHS, and in particular the U.S. Food and Drug Administration (FDA), a branch of DHHS, failed to follow some important aspects of the Commission's recommendations, discussed later in this chapter (also see Levine 1991), the Commission nevertheless had a valuable effect. At the time of its final meeting in 1978, its conclusions, entitled *The Belmont Report: Ethical Principles and Guidelines for the Protection of Human Subjects of Research* (National Commission for the Protection of Human Subjects 1979) were submitted. Although not directly codified in regulatory statutes, they did greatly influence the form of the federal regulations and the general ethical approach to be used with undertaking experimentation in human subjects. On a practical basis these concepts often do guide the day-to-day deliberations of the IRB. The three basic principles set forth in the Belmont Report are as follows (adapted from Levine 1991, pp. 14–18, and "Protecting Human Research Subjects" 1993, pp. xxi–xxiii):

1. **Respect for persons.**

   A person is entitled to choice, dignity, privacy, and confidentiality. This concept was stated by Emanuel Kant: "So act as to treat humanity, whether in thine own person or in that of any other, in every case as an end withal, never as a means only." Or, in the words of the Commission, "respect for persons incorporates at least two basic ethical convictions: first, that individuals should be treated as autonomous agents and second, that persons with diminished autonomy and thus need of protection are entitled to such protections" (Levine 1991, p. 15).

2. **Beneficence.**

   Maximize good/minimize harm. On a practical basis this means that the research effort is to be constructed so as to maximize the anticipated benefit to the subject while minimizing any foreseeable risks. In the words of the Commission, "The term, beneficence, is often understood to cover acts of kindness or charity that go beyond strict application. In this document, beneficence is understood in a stronger sense—as an obligation. Two general rules have been formulated as complementary expressions of beneficent in this sense: 1) do no harm, 2) maximize possible benefits and minimize possible harms" (Levine 1991, p. 15).

3. **Justice.**

   Justice requires that we treat persons fairly and that we give each person what he or she is due or owed. The philosophical underpinnings of the concepts of justice are complicated and beyond the scope of this text, but in a practical matter come down to the following: 1) there will be no exploitative or coercive recruitment of subjects, and 2) those bearing risk of a condition will have a right to participate in and reap benefits of research.

A Brief History of Biomedical Research: The Need for Increased Scrutiny

Before the twentieth century, physicians generally had little concept of the scientific method, and the few studies undertaken were seriously flawed. Instructive in this regard is Lind's 1753 comparative trial of "the most promising treatment for scurvy" (Pocock 1983). This study had 12 patients divided into 6 different treatment groups (otherwise controlled for diet and bunking in the same place on the ship); despite the obvious lack of statistical power, the 2 patients on the supplemental diet of oranges and lemons had the "most sudden and visible effects" in terms of recovery from their scurvy (the first returned to duty, the second became the other sailors' nurse). Nonetheless, Lind continued to propose "pure dry air" as the best treatment for scurvy, with fresh citrus fruit as the second choice. Another example of the physician's lack of consideration for the scientific method at that time is seen in Rush's report nearly 50 years later (1794), *On the Treatment of Yellow Fever by Bleedings*: "I began by drawing a small quantity at a time. The appearance of the blood and its effect upon the system satisfied me of its safety and efficacy. Never before did I experience such sublime joy as I now felt in contemplating the success of my remedies" (Pocock 1983, p. 15).

Before the 1930s there was little incentive to conduct properly designed trials. Although pharmaceutical companies did enjoy considerable growth after World War I, most of their compounds were plant derivatives; apart from insulin, penicillin, and the sulfonamides, few agents were added to the world's pharmacopoeia before the mid-1940s. With the passage of the Food, Drug and Cosmetic Act of 1938 ("Milestones in U.S. Food and Drug Law History" 1999), much of this situation changed. Although demonstration of drug efficacy in humans was still largely anecdotal, this legislation required that formal animal research be undertaken to test for drug toxicity. In the wake of the thalidomide problem that emerged in 1962, the Kefauver-Harris Drug Amendments required safety studies in humans and a more rigorous proof of efficacy ("Milestones" 1999). However, it was not until 1969 that FDA required evidence from randomized clinical trials to establish the efficacy of pharmaceuticals (Pocock 1983). The institution of these new regulations would lead to a large increase in the need for controlled clinical trials and eventually to the huge research and development industry in pharmacology that we see today. Since a large number of subjects were involved in that research, it follows that increased government scrutiny attended the efforts of the research industry.

Public Response to Unethical Research

Although both the huge sums of money expended and the large number of subjects being exposed to risks in studies doubtless contributed to increasing regulatory supervision, probably the most important factor in this regard was the public's perception that people were being exposed to unacceptable risks in the course of experimentation. Although public knowledge of unethical research did not come until late in the 1960s to the 1970s, it is instructional to look back to World War II to understand the direction that research took and the momentum that developed during that war and in the 20-plus years that followed.

In December 1941, President Roosevelt created the Committee on Medical Research (CMR) to coordinate the wartime medical research effort. In the course of the war the CMR expended some $25 million, involving 600 research proposals (Rothman 1991). Given the difficulties of undertaking research on soldiers in the battlefield, civilians were often used, usually without their knowledge or consent, to help with the wartime research effort. For example, at the Ohio Soldier and Sailors Orphanage a number of children were subjected to a vaccination trial against dysentery in which they were injected with killed suspensions of shigela. They invariably had severe local and systemic reactions, often with temperatures up to 104.6 degrees (Rothman 1991). At the Dickson Illinois Institute for the Retarded and at the New Jersey State Colony for the Feeble Minded, studies were undertaken to determine the efficacy of sulfonamide against dysentery. It was understood that the research carried significant dangers to the subjects, including extensive kidney damage and even death. There is no suggestion that the subjects or their relatives knew that these children were part of an experiment (Rothman 1991).

The deficiencies in the protection of research subjects were pointedly brought to the public eye in 1966 with the publication, in the *New England Journal of Medicine* (NEJM) of Henry Beecher's controversial article "Ethics in Clinical Research" (Beecher 1966). Beecher, then the Dorr Professor of Research in Anesthesia at Harvard Medical School, mentioned at the beginning of his article that an examination of 100 consecutive human studies published in 1964 in what he characterized as "an excellent journal" revealed that 12 of them seemed to be unethical. For the article he had originally compiled 50 examples of research involving questionable ethics; in only 2 of these studies was consent mentioned. In the final NEJM version he provided 22 examples (the list was shortened for publication) of research published in respected journals by prominent researchers that had involved very significant risks to nonconsenting research subjects. This article makes for some very compelling reading.

The response of the public, and that of its representatives in Congress, was quite significant (Beecher had notified the press in advance of the publication). Further, Beecher's article was published at about the same time that Dr. Chester Southam was coming under significant public criticism for his research involving the injection of live cancer cells into elderly, senile patients without their knowledge (Rothman 1991).

In light of these disclosures, significant public pressure was brought to bear on the National Institutes of Health (NIH) to regulate those involved in biomedical research. During 1966, NIH established guidelines covering all federally funded research involving human experimentation. With these guidelines, calling for review by a "committee of institutional associates" (Levine 1991), we see the beginnings of the IRB.

Several more examples of unethical medical research came to public attention. Perhaps most notable among these was the Tuskegee Syphilis Study, which ran from 1932 until 1972, when it came under intense public scrutiny. The research involved 400 black men with syphilis and approximately 200 black men without syphilis who served as control subjects. The study was intended to clarify the issue of whether the treatments available at the time, such as heavy metals and arsenic, could be adding to the neurological complications of syphilis. The patients were recruited without knowledge of their condition (often being told they had "bad blood") and were told that the investigative procedures (such as spinal taps) were in actuality "special free treatment." After 4 years it was apparent that those in the untreated group had many more complications, and within 10 years it was ascertained that the death rate in the infected subjects was about twice as high as in the control subjects. When penicillin became available in the late 1940s, the subjects were not offered this effective treatment despite the evidence that the syphilis shortened their life span by about 20%. The study continued until 1972, when accounts of it appeared in the national press (Levine 1991, pp. 69–70; Rothman 1991, p. 82).

The fact that many of these studies involved mostly impoverished minorities was not well received by the public during that time of increasing interest in civil rights. In 1968, Walter Mondale, then a senator from Minnesota, introduced a bill to establish a commission, to be titled the Commission on Health Science and Society, to study the social and ethical implications of advances in the biomedical field (Rothman 1991). Although a number of congressional hearings were held, Mondale was not successful in establishing a commission. At about this time, considerable public attention was drawn to a baby with Down's syndrome and an intestinal defect who had been allowed to starve to death at Johns Hopkins University Hospital (Rothman 1991). Similar cases concerning the seriously medically ill, as well as increasing public concern over the ethics of transplant and the research cases cited previously, increased public pressure for some regulation of the biomedical field. Mondale, disturbed by the cavalier attitude regarding ethical concerns exhibited by transplant surgeons in the 1968 hearings, persisted in his efforts to establish a commission. As Tuskegee came to public attention in 1972, Mondale was joined in his efforts by Senators Edward Kennedy and Jacob Javits; their combined efforts resulted in the establishment of the Commission in 1974, along with other legislation that is discussed below (Rothman 1991).

Recent Federal Regulations and Current Administration of the Institutional Review Board

The Surgeon General, under significant external pressure, directed in 1966 that all Public Health Service (PHS) grants should have some committee review. In 1974, DHEW (overseeing PHS) issued regulations that more formally established the human subjects committee by stipulating the number and composition of its membership, as well as further clarifying its duties. These rules were codified in the Code of Federal Regulations (CFR) Title 45, Part 46 (from here on referred to as 45 CFR 46). (For all CFR titles cited in this chapter, see "Federal Policy for the Protection of Human Subjects" 1991; or see Appendix E for the CFR Web site.) Significant revisions of DHEW regulations were undertaken by both NIH and FDA in 1981 (in response to the Commission's recommendations) and again in 1991 (to coordinate the regulatory efforts of the 16 federal agencies involved in human subjects research) (Levine 1991). The regulations most germane to clinical research efforts are covered by NIH's 45 CFR 46. Similar regulations are codified by FDA under Title 21, parts 50 and 56 (part 50 is concerned with the elements of informed consent–also covered by 45 CFR 46). Since FDA regulates both drugs and medical devices, there are additional statutes that reflect this mandate: part 312 (Investigational New Drug Application), part 812 (Investigational Device Exemptions), and part 860 (Medical Device Classification Procedures).

One may wonder why two federal agencies have so much overlap in their regulatory efforts. Indeed, so did both the Commission (1974–1978) and the President's Commission (1980–1983); they had recommended that all administration of federal regulations involving research on human subjects be established in a single office. The FDA was explicitly identified as one of the offices to be subsumed under this office (Levine 1991), but even before the Commission had issued its final report (the Belmont Report), FDA had announced in 1978 its intention of not following this legislative mandate (Levine 1991). Therefore there currently exists the unfortunate situation that the IRB's functioning and much clinical research are overseen by two agencies. Currently, protocols are subject to review under both FDA and NIH regulations; both sets of regulations apply, and the requirements of both sets of regulations must be met ("Protecting Human Research Subjects" 1993).

The Office for Protection From Research Risks (OPRR) is the branch of NIH that administers the regulatory functions protecting human subjects in research (via 45 CFR 46). As we have seen, NIH has a long history of supporting biomedical research in an effort to address a number of public health problems. On the other hand, FDA is primarily a regulatory agency that concerns itself with overseeing the purity of drugs and assuring the lack of adulterants in foods. This mission dates back to the Drug Importation Act of 1848, when the U.S. Customs worked against importation of adulterated drugs ("Milestones" 1999). As a regulatory agency, FDA acts as such in its inspection of research projects; as Levine states, in site visits to IRBs, rather than the colleagues and experts one expects from NIII, FDA will appear with badges, presenting "Notices of Inspection" that "look for all the world like search warrants. . . . FDA's approach reflects its history as an agency having as one of its major functions the detection of miscreants" (Levine 1991, p. 358).

For the most part, 45 CFR 46 will serve as a guide to our discussion of the current regulations regarding research involving human subjects. Aside from work with medical devices, FDA's regulatory statutes do not come into play until one gets into trouble (a topic discussed near the end of this chapter).

In accordance with generally held "ethical norms" (Levine 1991), the IRB follows a basic framework in reviewing each project, including consideration of the following:

1. The rights and welfare of the individual(s) involved

2. The appropriateness of the methods used to secure informed consent

3. The balance of risks and potential benefits of the investigation

In carrying out this mandate, the IRB, although working within the constraints of various federal regulations, is not just an enforcer of these regulations or a direct intermediary of the government. Rather, the IRB is an agent of its own institution (Levine 1991, p. 342), guided not only by the minimal standards of the federal rules but also by ethical concerns and its own judgment to provide for the institution that it serves. Indeed, in many cases these review committees were active at their institutions before being legislated into existence by the USPHS. An IRB that justifies its decisions with "we are just following the statutes" rather than citing its own authority and judgment is not doing its job. OPRR requires that each institution must provide a "statement of principles governing the institution in . . . protecting the rights and welfare of" human research subjects (Levine 1991, p. x; 45 CFR 46.103). This implies a degree of autonomy for the committee in ensuring the welfare of research subjects within the institution.

Composition of the Institutional Review Board

It is stated in 45 CFR 46.107 that "each IRB shall have at least five members, with varying backgrounds to promote complete and adequate review of research activities commonly conducted by the institution." Also mandated is a diversity of the members in regard to race, gender, and cultural background. No IRB may consist of members from entirely one profession, and each IRB is required to have one member not affiliated with the institution (often labeled the community member). "If an IRB regularly reviews research that involves a vulnerable category of subjects, such as children, prisoners, pregnant women, or handicapped or mentally disabled persons, consideration shall be given to the inclusion of one or more individuals who are knowledgeable about and experienced in working with these subjects."

Informed Consent

Generating a good consent form is probably one of the most important aspects of one's interaction with the IRB; not providing one is likely to result in delays in the approval process in the form of stipulations. As will be discussed, there are a number of resources available to help one with the necessary elements of writing a good consent, but as an exercise we will first present an "improper" consent form, with some annotations suggesting improvements. This form begins on the next page.

As indicated above, the writing of proper consent forms is of utmost importance; many IRB members are compulsive in their examination of the consent forms that come before them and tend to focus on small defects in the document. It is with this IRB focus in mind that Levine (1991) observes, "I believe that there is no more expensive or less competent redaction service available in the United States than that provided by an alarmingly large number of IRB's" (p. 326). What Levine is expressing is the importance of focusing on the *process* of informed consent, not merely on getting the form signed. The informed-consent process entails ongoing discussion with the research subject, answering questions, clarifying issues of risks versus benefits, and providing the subject with information as the study proceeds.

Nonetheless, you also need to learn how to write good consent forms. In 45 CFR 46.116, you can read the "General Requirements for Informed Consent," but your IRB is probably your best source of information. Many IRBs are now providing helpful informational packets along with the application forms. These packets usually contain a checklist to assure the completeness of the application, along with a review concerning the elements of informed consent, and even a fill-in-the-blank sample of a consent form (many IRBs have apparently tired of being an editing service).

Following the incorrect consent form is a correct consent form, rewritten to include the necessary elements that were commented on in the incorrect form.

Precautions in Working With the Mentally Ill

There are several aspects of our "Remit" study sample forms that necessitate further discussion. First, the study involves schizophrenic patients, who are potentially vulnerable subjects and potentially not competent to provide informed consent. Second, this is a placebo-controlled trial, which brings up difficulties still being addressed by the OPRR. We discuss the difficulties of working with the vulnerable mentally ill first.

The Potentially Impaired Subject

In its directive to the IRBs for approval requirements, 45 CFR 46.111 states the expectation that "when some or all of the subjects are likely to be vulnerable to coercion or undue influence, such as children, prisoners, pregnant

Incorrect Consent Form

Consent Form for Schizophrenia Study	Comments regarding the form
You are invited to participate in a randomized, placebo controlled trial of a new drug for the treatment of schizophrenia. You are being asked if you would be willing to participate in the study, since you are currently hospitalized for schizophrenia at _____ Hospital.	The consent form needs to be written in simple language without technical jargon. "Randomized" (like the flip of a coin) and "placebo" (like a sugar pill) need to be defined, as well as "placebo controlled."
Please read the information that follows and decide whether or not you would like to participate in this study.	The investigators doing the study should be identified in the introductory paragraph. Source of funding needs to be identified.
This is a randomized, placebo-controlled trial of a new drug to treat schizophrenia. The drug is named "Remit." This is a drug that has been shown to help some patients, but in the current study we intend to find out whether it helps most patients who receive it by controlling for the effects of a placebo. If you agree to be in this study you will be assigned randomly to receive either the drug "Remit" or placebo for the first 2 weeks of your hospitalization at _____ Hospital.	This consent is quite jumbled; it is best to first present background information explaining the purpose of the study, then describe the procedures to be followed by the subject while in the study: this covers frequency of questionnaires, blood draws, physical examinations, and the length of the study.
At the end of that time the investigators responsible for the study will "break the blind" to see which medication you have been receiving. If you have been responding to the medication you have been receiving (Remit or placebo), you can continue on that drug for an additional 2 weeks, or if you are not improving you can be switched to an alternative drug at that time.	Need to explain that an experimental drug is being used; in addition, if there are no benefits to being in the study (as with this one), this should be stated.
You will receive the medication at the end of each day in pill form prior to going to bed.	
Remit is generally a very safe medication that sometimes causes dry mouth and blurred vision and has been associated with some neurological problems. However, these are fairly uncommon and you should do fine on the medication. We really don't anticipate any serious problems.	Expected frequency of side effects should be mentioned and defined; "neurological problems" is too vague a term.

(continued)

Need to discuss alternatives to being in the study (including other treatments that may more clearly benefit the subject).

If you sign up for the study but later change your mind and decide you don't want to participate, you can drop from the study without any adverse consequences and will be allowed to continue in the hospital.

What is a rating instrument? (Avoid technical jargon.) Need to explain or emphasize that "detailed questions" may be of a sensitive nature. Should be in the "risks" section.

This information should be in the section on what the subject will be expected to do (near the beginning of the consent form).

If you are in the study, we will periodically assess you using a rating instrument that will ask you detailed questions about your symptoms. This will be administered 3 times a week. Other than this, your treatment on the ward will be the same as other patients'.

This statement should be combined with the information two paragraphs above. Emphasize the voluntary nature of participation and ability to withdraw without affecting future relationships with the investigators or their cooperating institutions.

Discuss precautions taken to assure confidentiality, and warn that confidentiality is not absolute, because there will be monitoring by the FDA or the drug company sponsoring the study. There needs to be an out-of-study contact in case of questions about the study. Often, the hospital's patient relations department will agree to do this.

You are making a decision whether or not to participate. If you decide to participate, you are free to withdraw at any time without prejudice. You will not be identified in any publications that result from this study and only aggregate data will be presented.

If the subject has a guardian, there needs to be space for that (along with the guardian's relationship to the patient).

Your signature below indicates that you have decided to participate. Please contact Dr. _____ at _____ (phone) if you have any further questions later.

Thank you for your consideration.

Signature of Patient _____

Date _____

Consent Form

Double-Blind, Placebo-Controlled Study for the Investigational Drug Remit in the Treatment of Chronic Schizophrenia

You are invited to be in a research study looking at a new drug being investigated for treatment of the chronic mental illness known as schizophrenia. The study will attempt to discover how well this new drug works. You were selected as a possible participant because you have been diagnosed as having schizophrenia. We ask that you read this form and ask any questions you may have before agreeing to be in the study.

The study is being conducted by Dr. X and Dr. Y in the Department of Psychiatry at Z hospital.

Background Information

The purpose of this study is to determine whether the experimental drug Remit might be effective in the treatment of schizophrenia. The Feeling Good Pharmaceutical Company, which is the manufacturer of this drug and the sponsor of this current research study, is in the process of obtaining the approval of the U.S. Food and Drug Administration (FDA) for the use of this medication in schizophrenia. The efficacy (effectiveness) of the drug will be looked at in individuals who have had a diagnosis of schizophrenia for at least one year and whose condition has worsened to the extent that they require hospitalization.

Procedures

If you agree to be in this study, we would ask you to do the following things:

First, it is hoped that you will be able to remain in the hospital for at least two weeks, which is the duration of the first part the study.

Soon after your hospitalization you will be assessed for your suitability for the study with an extensive psychiatric interview, which may last as long as two to three hours.

Throughout the remainder of the hospitalization you will be scheduled for interviews, occurring three times a week and each lasting approximately 30 minutes, which will ask about your psychiatric symptoms as well as possible side effects from the medications that you are receiving.

This study has what is called a double-blind, placebo-controlled design. This means that you will be assigned to receive either active study medication (in this case, Remit) or a placebo (like an inactive sugar pill). Whether you receive the active drug or placebo will be determined in a random fashion (like a flip of a coin). "Double-blind" means that neither you or the investigators doing this study will know whether you are receiving the active drug or the placebo. In this case your chances of receiving the active drug are two in three.

Also, we will be asking you for a blood sample to be drawn, amounting to approximately one tablespoon of blood, three times: at the beginning of this study, at the end of the first week, and at the end of the second week.

(continued)

Risks and Benefits of Being in the Study

The study has several risks.

- First, you may end up in the placebo group, in which case you will not be receiving the study medication to help your condition.
- Second, the psychiatric interviews do involve our asking some personal questions that you might find threatening or confusing. However, you are free to decline to answer these questions at any time throughout the interview.
- Third, the study medication does have a potential for side effects. As many as 1 in 10 patients have dry mouth and blurred vision or some stiffness in their muscles. Another potential complication of taking the medication is a condition known as tardive dyskinesia, which results in involuntary movement in the muscles of the face or other parts of your body. This condition has not been encountered in those using this specific drug, but it has been previously seen in those taking drugs of this class of tranquilizers, so it remains a possibility in your case.
- Last, there may be some bruising or discomfort in the area where the blood is drawn.

The benefits to participation in this study are that you may have a good response to the study medication and see an improvement in your condition.

You will receive no cash payments for being involved in this study.

Alternatives to Participating in This Study

As an alternative to being in this study, you can receive medications that currently have FDA approval for treatment of your mental illness.

Compensation

If this research activity results in an injury, treatment will be available, including first aid, emergency treatment, and follow-up care as needed. Payment for any such treatment must be provided by you or your third-party payer, if any (health insurance, Medicare, etc.).

You will not be charged for the psychiatric care or blood testing that occurs during your hospitalization, and the pharmaceutical company sponsoring this study has agreed to pay for the excess days you might spend in the hospital in order to complete the two weeks of the study.

Confidentiality

The records of this study will be kept private. In any sort of report we might publish, we will not include any information that will make it possible to identify a subject. Your record for the study may, however, be reviewed by the drug manufacturer or by representatives of the FDA. To that extent, confidentiality isn't absolute.

(continued)

Voluntary Nature of the Study

Your decision whether or not to participate will not affect your current or future relations with the Z University. If you decide to participate, you are free to withdraw at any time without affecting those relationships.

New Information

If, during the course of this research study, there are significant new findings discovered that might influence your willingness to continue, the researchers will inform you of those findings.

Contacts and Questions

The researchers conducting this study are Drs. X and Y. You may ask any questions you have now. If you have questions later, you may contact them at phone number xxx-xxxx. Or, you may contact the Patient Relations Department at Z Hospital at phone number yyy-yyyy.

You will be given a copy of this form to keep for your records.

Statement of Consent

I have read the above information. I have asked questions and have received answers. I consent to participate in the study.

Signature _____

Date _____

Signature of Investigator _____

Date _____

women, mentally disabled persons, or economically or educationally disadvantaged persons, *additional safeguards* [italics added] have been included in the study to protect the rights and welfare of these subjects." As will be discussed later in this chapter, the OPRR is quite explicit about the safeguards that need to be in place to protect children, prisoners, and pregnant women, but much less so concerning the "mentally disabled." Because of the great spectrum in patients' functioning, schizophrenia in itself is not a condition that leads automatically to an inability to participate in the consent process. Likewise, the concepts of competence or incompetence (being primarily legal constructs) are not particularly helpful here. The issue is more one of comprehension by the potential subjects. Several studies have shown that hospitalized psychiatric patients (most with schizophrenia) are equal to the medically ill in their understanding of a research protocol, but there are some studies at variance with this finding (Appelbaum 1996). The use of a guardian or proxy (although in certain situations this approach can be useful) is controversial because of significant pitfalls. Whereas a proxy's consent might be necessary if a patient is to receive a medical treatment—where there is an expected benefit with a medically acknowledged risk—different factors are operating in entering a research study, where one must assume a certain risk for altruistic reasons; this must be a personal choice. Although potentially vulnerable populations will be exposed to the hazards of research, the OPRR is mindful of the importance of continuing psychiatric research because of the potential benefits to the subject population as a whole. A parallel line of argument is seen in the regulation that allows research in children involving more than minimal risk if it "is likely to yield generalizable knowledge about the subjects' disorder or condition that is of vital importance for the understanding or amelioration of the subjects' disorder or condition" (45 CFR 46.406c).

The Placebo Problem

In undertaking placebo-controlled studies, similar precautions are called for in the consent process and monitoring of the patient. We are reminded of this in considering a study undertaken by researchers at UCLA Medical School in which several research subjects had adverse outcomes, including one suicide. In response to complaints against the researchers, the OPRR issued a report of its findings in May 1994 (Applebaum 1996). The controversy was also widely covered by the popular media, congressional hearings were held, and a lawsuit was brought by the family of one of the subjects.

This important study involved a group of schizophrenic patients who were followed on a fixed dose of Prolixin Decanoate (fluphenazine decanoate) for 1 year and then, after a withdrawal protocol, randomized to Prolixin versus placebo for up to 1 year, or until psychotic relapse occurred. The study was looking into the predictors of successful functioning exclusive of neuroleptic medication (Appelbaum 1996). The OPRR found that the monitoring of the patients was acceptable. However, fault was found with the informed-consent process and with the clinicians' not being clear that they were also acting as investigators. Indeed, one of the research subjects (later turned plaintiff) was quoted as saying he was delighted to get into the research program "because I thought I was going to get the premier treatment, while they did a little research on the side" (Applebaum 1996, p. 4).

There are significant potential ethical pitfalls to be considered in the use of placebo control groups, particularly in psychiatric populations. Indeed, the Declaration of Helsinki (see Appendix B, this volume) states: "In any medical study, every patient—including those of a control group, if any—should be assured of the best proven diagnostic and therapeutic method" (II, 3). However, progress in research, and particularly the demonstration of the efficacy of new drugs, demands placebo-controlled trials (and FDA has a strong preference for them). This area is one of active debate, thankfully, beyond the reach of concrete regulation—and one that often consumes the best energies of the IRBs. One can expect quite variable responses from the IRBs, but it is hoped that one can also expect some consistency in the approval of studies that are mindful of the consent, monitoring, and risk/benefit concerns.

Of practical importance to be considered in the placebo-controlled study, and in the use of investigational drugs in general, is the role of the third-party payer. A growing number of insurance companies, particularly in managed care, will not pay for drug therapy intended for investigational use. None would knowingly pay for an inpatient's participation in a placebo-controlled trial (as in our "Remit" study, on preceding pages).

Developments in recent years could significantly change the way we approach working with potentially vulnerable populations, particularly in the area of placebo-controlled trials. In December 1998 the National Bioethics Advisory Committee (NBAC) issued a report entitled *Research Involving Persons With Mental Illness That May Affect Decisionmaking Capacity* (National Bioethics Advisory Committee 1998). The NBAC was appointed by President Clinton in 1995 to review U.S. federal protections pertaining to human subject research (Woodward 1999). A number of controversial recommendations were made in this sizable document, including the requirement that a patient with mental illness or a family member of such a patient serve on the IRB and that an independent, qualified professional assess the research subject's capacity to consent. The NBAC report has generated a great deal of controversy within the psychiatric community (Charney et al. 1999; Oldham et al. 1999).

The local IRBs have been under increased pressure from OPRR regarding their regulatory mandate. During late 1998 through 1999, research activities have been restricted or suspended at eight institutions by OPRR as a result of perceived shortcomings in oversight by their IRBs. Inadequate protection of vulnerable subjects and failure of the investigators to assess risks in consent forms accurately were the most common complaints cited (Woodward 1999). These actions by OPRR have garnered a great deal of attention by the popular media as well.

Clearly, with all this activity from the NBAC and OPRR, there will probably be a formal response in the form of new federal regulations regarding the way research is conducted on psychiatric populations.

Prisoners

Because of the circumstances of their incarceration, prisoners are thought to be in need of special protection because of the problems inherent in "their ability to make a truly voluntary and uncoerced decision whether or not to participate as subjects in research" (45 CFR 46.302). In consideration of their potential vulnerability, significant restrictions are in place regarding the type of research that may be done on the prison population. There are a number of provisions that ensure a lack of coercion (related to sentences, living conditions, and so forth) in recruitment of subjects. In addition, the majority of the IRB members must have no affiliation with the prison, and there must be at least one prisoner on the committee. More important, the research may involve only minimal risk or be limited to areas such as "conditions particularly affecting prisoners" or "study of the possible causes, effects, and processes of incarceration, and of criminal behavior" (45 CFR 46.306). This research may proceed only after approval by the secretary of DHHS in consultation with experts in that field and a published notice in the Federal Register of the intent to pursue this research.

Equitable Selection of Subjects

Throughout much of this chapter we have focused on the negative aspects of undertaking research, in consideration either of the risks to the subjects or of the cost to society in general (related to the substantial NIH budget). These risks and costs are assumed in the hope that the research will potentially benefit our society as a whole and that the findings will be generalized to as large a segment of the population as feasible. This sentiment is now reflected in regulations that require that researchers make an equitable selection of subjects from a diverse group of potential subjects while remaining cognizant of the needs of special populations (45 CFR 46.110). Therefore, one needs to design a study with a wide range of ages, without regard to race and being careful not to exclude women of childbearing potential. Before 1993, FDA had restricted women of childbearing age from entering Phase 1 and Phase 2 trials of drug and biological agents. However, since the publication of the "Guidelines for the Study and Evaluation of Gender Differences in the Clinical Evaluation of Drugs" (1993) by FDA in the Federal Register, the participation of women of childbearing age has been encouraged. Pregnancy testing is recommended as part of the protocol, and women must be counseled to use a reliable method of contraception while participating in the clinical trial (FDA Information Sheets for Institutional Review Boards and Clinic Investigators 1995). However, pregnant women are not as a class to be excluded from studies, particularly if the information to be gained during the study could be of interest or benefit to this group. In reconsidering the previous guidelines and concluding that they should be revised, the agency stated that it felt that "this does not reflect a lack of concern for potential exposure or indifference to potential fetal damage, but rather the agency's opinion that 1) exclusion of women from early trials is not medically necessary because the risk of fetal exposure can be minimized by patient behavior and laboratory testing, and 2) initial determinations about whether that risk is adequately addressed are properly left to patients, physicians, local IRBs, and sponsors, with appropriate review and guidance by FDA, as are all other aspects of the safety of proposed investigations" ("Guidelines" 1993).

Getting Into Trouble

The text of 45 CFR 46.113 reads: "An IRB shall have authority to suspend or terminate approval of research that is not being conducted in accordance with the IRB's requirements or that has been associated with unexpected serious harm to subjects." The regulation goes on to state the necessity for the IRB to mention the causes for action and also notify appropriate institutional officials and the department or agency head. In some cases the action may have been brought in response to some unanticipated adverse event or may have been the result of some benign misunderstanding involving one of the subjects or some aspect of the protocol. In these cases the matter can be settled informally between the investigator and the IRB. However, if the violations demonstrate a disregard for protection of human subjects or serious noncompliance, the IRB and the administrative structure within the institution will be obligated to notify FDA and OPRR. According to "FDA Information Sheets" (1995), "FDA may disqualify clinical investigators from receiving investigational drugs only when the investigator has repeatedly or deliberately violated the Agency's regulations, or has submitted false information to the sponsor in a required report" (p. 93). The FDA upon hearing of the matter will then notify the investigator of an "informal conference" (Warning Letter) which calls for a timely response that could settle the matter. If there is a significant violation involved, the proceedings continue through a Hearing for Proposed Disqualification and then a Final Order on Disqualification, which involves some degree of public disclosure. Criminal prosecution is always a possibility for those "clinical investigators who have knowingly or willingly submitted false information to a research sponsor" ("FDA Information Sheets" 1995, p. 97).

Practical Pointers for Working With the Institutional Review Board

1. Do not be intimidated or threatened, and try not to get angry, but do ask questions. Working with IRBs can be frustrating. Remember that you and the IRB have the same basic goals and that most members are scientists like you. The IRB is sometimes as confused by the current regulations as you are (the regulations are always in flux), but the IRB in general knows more than you do about them.

2. Keep track of the number of subjects you have enrolled in the study. If you run over the limit that you asked for at the time of application (and this is easy to do), you cannot use the data from these subjects (since they are not approved), and you are in violation of FDA and OPRR rules.

3. There is nothing to be gained by being condescending or sarcastic in your interactions with the IRB. You might be upset (perhaps justifiably) by the committee's criticism of a proposal for a project, but there is nothing to be gained by a heated reply.

4. If you have an ethically difficult project (with consent problems in a vulnerable population, possible problems with placebo control, and so forth), it is a good idea to approach one of the administrative staff of the IRB for help. He or she can refer you to a committee member with interests in this area.

5. Likewise, the administrative staff can often be of immense help in answering procedural questions such as how to fill out forms, in informing you when your proposal is to go before the committee, and in like matters.

6. The best way to learn about the IRB is to become a member. It will also give you much experience in research methodology and keep you abreast of ongoing research in your institution.

Conclusion

The nature of medical practice has changed much over the last 50 years, especially within the context of the doctor-patient relationship, and a number of third parties have become involved in the interaction. Governmental involvement in the relationship between researcher and subject has also grown significantly during this period. Many of these developments appear to have occurred in response to the realization that performing research on patients creates unique stresses on this relationship. Often there is money, prestige, or promotion to be gained in getting the project done, and the various demands on one's time may suggest to one the need or desirability to bend the rules a bit. It is important, early in one's career, to appreciate—or at least reconcile oneself to—the fact that IRBs are a significant, necessary, useful part of the life of a clinical researcher. When you approach IRBs with such a mindset, they become part of your research program.

It is also important to remember that research involving other people does generate an unequal interchange: the researcher is in charge. In looking at the past, we see that much research has been done that we must now consider unethical, although there is nothing to be gained by judging too harshly those who worked in earlier years. Instead, it is important to remember that competent researchers in the past have made human-subject research decisions that did not hold up under public scrutiny. IRBs now provide the scrutiny for us. We now find ourselves living with a set of rules to guide us in the process of our research. Although it is impossible to regulate ethical behavior, many of the rules under which we operate do help to provide protection for our patients or for other individuals who are willing to be our research subjects. Experience has taught us that outside scrutiny is essential, and we should not only tolerate this scrutiny but also seek it and welcome it, realizing that it is an important part of the process of conducting ethical research.

CHAPTER 9

Ethics and Misconduct

In Chapter 8, we were primarily concerned with the ethical conduct of *research* and the regulatory oversight governing this endeavor as it relates to the protection of research subjects in their interaction with the investigator. In this chapter, we focus on the expected behavior of the investigator concerning the handling of data, publishing of material, and relating to coauthors and industrial sponsors. Within this literature, numerous debates have resulted in significant change from a regulatory perspective. As such, a comprehensive review of the subject is beyond the scope of this chapter. Instead, we attempt to inform the new investigator about certain issues with a series of practical "ethical scenarios" that illustrate ethical concerns that may arise in the course of a clinical study. We also discuss a recent case of alleged scientific misconduct that received much media attention so as to illustrate both the public's and the scientific community's interest in this area and the ongoing difficulties that are encountered in addressing these cases.

In the conclusion of Chapter 8, we alluded to the pressures on the researcher to perhaps overlook the rights of their subjects so as to expedite the study process. These pressures do not end when the data have been collected. The researcher is still confronted with the rigors of analyzing the information, writing it up, and finding a venue in which to publish the results. The researcher is expected to proceed through this sequence in an ethical manner and not be tempted to trim data, unnecessarily break up the material to maximize the number of publications, or engage in other types of unethical behavior on the route to publication. However, because of substantial internal and external pressures, unethical behavior may occur during this process. Research is a great deal of work, and the direct reward is the publication. Advancing through the academic ranks, being awarded grants and tenure, and even being able to continue with one's research are predicated on the ability of the researcher to publish. This situation may bring considerable stress on the ethical comportment of the investigator, a fact not lost on the funding entities, the publishers of scientific journals, or the regulatory bodies involved in overseeing research. And unfortunately it appears that all these parties have cause for concern.

The precursors of such problems may be manifested long before one's research career in clinical psychiatry begins. Petersdorf (1986), in his article "The Pathogenesis of Fraud in Medical Science," talked of the "premed syndrome" and how the rigors of competition for medical education lead to cheating. He cited a study of 400 medical students at Chicago medical schools that found that 88% of the students reported having cheated as premedical students and that these students frequently endorsed agreement with statements such as "people have to cheat in this dog-eat-dog world."

We discuss some of the work being done to address such problems after we present a highly publicized case of alleged scientific misconduct. This case serves to demonstrate how badly things can go wrong in investigating problems of scientific conduct and to illustrate the imperfect mechanisms in place for addressing allegations of impropriety in research. We then discuss one author's construct of "the spectrum of ethical offenses," followed by some ethical scenarios to illustrate these concepts.

Problems With an Article in the Journal *Cell*

On June 21, 1996, an appeals panel of the U.S. Department of Health and Human Services (DHHS) cleared Thereza Imanishi-Kari, Ph.D., of 19 charges of scientific misconduct, concluding that "the preponderance of the evidence" did not support the government case against her (Kaiser and Marshall 1996, p. 1864). This decision came after 6 weeks of hearings and deliberations involving some 70 original laboratory notebooks and 6,500 pages of transcripts from the hearings. This appeals panel overturned a 1994 ruling by the Office of Research Integrity (ORI) that recommended Imanishi-Kari be barred from receiving federal research funds for an unprecedented 10-year period. The ORI decision was the result of 5 years of deliberation. However, the dispute goes back still further and involves much more than a (then) junior researcher who reported subsequently disputed results in a publication.

The case originates with an article (Weaver et al. 1986) about the production of antibodies in transgenic mice that was written by Imanishi-Kari with the Nobel laureate David Baltimore, Ph.D., as a coauthor. In 1985, a postdoctoral research fellow, Margot O'Toole, Ph.D., accused Imanishi-Kari of fraud when she was unable to replicate some of the original research results and insisted that the article be corrected. Baltimore and Imanishi-Kari rigorously denied wrongdoing and refused to correct the article. Subsequent investigations at the Massachusetts Institute of Technology, where the original work was done, and then at Tufts University, where Imanishi-Kari had become an assistant professor, failed to find any evidence of misconduct.

Because of persistent pressure by O'Toole and others (Kevles 1996), a special panel of the National Institutes of Health (NIH) became involved in 1988. Although errors were found that were significant enough to call for correction, fraud or scientific misconduct was not found (Marwick 1996).

However, in 1989, Congressman John Dingell (D, Mich), then chair of the Energy and Commerce Committee, decided to make this a test case to demonstrate the scientific community's inability to govern its members in cases of scientific misconduct. Dingell called for congressional hearings in 1988, 1989, and 1990 (resulting in some heated exchanges with Baltimore) and had the Secret Service do forensic analysis of Iminishi-Kari's notebooks for evidence of tampering. Because of all this activity, the NIH reopened its investigation, and the ORI (which had been formed at Dingell's insistence to identify scientific misconduct) became involved.

In 1991, an initial draft of the ORI's findings were leaked to the press. This document accused Imanishi-Kari of fraud and seriously discredited Baltimore, calling his persistent defense of his colleague "difficult to comprehend," while calling O'Toole's actions "heroic" (Kevles 1996, p. 107). Under significant pressure, Baltimore retracted his coauthorship of the *Cell* paper and resigned as president of Rockefeller University. In 1992, Baltimore withdrew the *Cell* paper retraction after United States prosecutors decided not to pursue criminal charges against Imanishi-Kari because jurors "were clearly incapable of understanding" the case (Anderson and Watson 1992, p. 177). After what Baltimore characterized as "a decade in limbo" (Kaiser and Marshall 1996), and great personal cost to Baltimore and Imanishi-Kari, these two researchers were finally cleared by the appeal board's decision.

This case involving mouse antibodies may seem to be a bit far afield from the area of clinical research in psychiatry. However, it does illustrate the intense governmental and media interest that can develop in this area and highlights current inadequacies in the administrative response to such allegations. This case also exemplifies the very difficult position in which the whistle-blower can find himself or herself. Initially, O'Toole was regarded as simply a nuisance, perhaps a disgruntled researcher with a gripe. The appeals board called O'Toole's interpretations of some events "improbable and unwarranted" and parts of her testimony "not credible" (Steele 1996). In contrast, those on the other side of the issue (the ORI and Dingell) called O'Toole's actions "heroic."

Spectrum of Ethical Offenses

The case described immediately above involved an allegation of fraud in its most blatant form: the faking of data. Scientific misconduct, however, usually involves less onerous transgressions and presumably those that are less deliberate. A good framework for defining the spectrum of fraud in science is provided in Dr. Marcia Angell's article "Editors and Fraud" (Angell 1983), in which she described the "seven stations" along the spectrum of scientific misconduct. As an editor of the *New England Journal of Medicine,* she has been very active in identifying the dynamics of the "publish or perish" situation and explaining what to do about it from the perspective of the editor; some of these suggestions are discussed in the conclusion of this chapter.

The seven stations, ranging from the most "benign" to the most "malignant," are summarized as follows; quoted material is from Angell (1983) (for the complete discussion of the seven stations, see p. 4):

1. *Fragmentation:* dividing a single study into "least publishable units" to maximize the number of articles generated

2. *Loose authorship:* The inclusion in papers of the names of coauthors who have not made significant contributions to the effort

3. *Duplication of publication:* publishing essentially the same study in more than one journal

4. *Selection of data:* presenting those data that conform to the hypothesis while ignoring those that do not

5. *Trimming:* actually changing numbers to conform to the hypothesis (a "more blatant way of dealing with unwelcome results")

6. *Plagiarism:* presenting the ideas or words of another as one's own (paraphrased from Merriam-Webster's Collegiate Dictionary, 10th ed.)

7. *Fabrication:* creating "an entire body of data, not just the alteration of isolated inconvenient results"

In the more malignant cases, such as fabrication, the act is usually deliberate, presumably fueled by the investigator's need for self-advancement. Plagiarism also can be the result of a deliberate act or an unfortunate oversight (an author always must be on his or her guard to avoid it). On the other hand, much of the behavior seen at the more benign end of the spectrum may result from either inadequate mentoring or a lack of education in the normative behavior expected of an ethical researcher. Accordingly, we present a few "ethical scenarios" to illustrate some situations that might arise early on in a research career.

Ethical Scenarios

These scenarios are the result of exchanges among the authors as well as material from the Association of American Medical Colleges' handbook for instructors titled *Teaching the Responsible Conduct of Research Through a Case Study Approach* (Korenman and Shipp 1994).

Loose Authorship

You are a psychiatric resident who is doing a small pilot outpatient trial of a medication that you think might be valuable for patients with a certain diagnosis. You are doing the entire protocol on your own. One of the faculty members, Dr. Smith, has helped you to develop the project, choose the instruments to administer, and obtain the necessary funding from your department for this pilot study. Dr. Jones, who is not involved in the project in any other way, has allowed you access to clinic space in the evenings to do the project. Dr. Smith will help you write up the results and prepare the data for publication. Should Dr. Smith be included as a coauthor on the publication that results from the study? Should Dr. Jones?

Ambiguous assignment of authorship is an issue that has created significant problems in the scientific community and is particularly vexing to journal editors. In an editorial to the *New England Journal of Medicine,* Kassirer and Angell (1991) mentioned a 12-page publication that listed 155 physicians from 63 institutions; the acknowledgments were 5 pages long. Adequate use of limited journal space is certainly a significant problem, but of more importance is that authorship should communicate something meaningful because it has so much to do with advancement in one's field. Accordingly, the International Committee of Medical Journal Editors published "Uniform Re quirements for Manuscripts Submitted to Biomedical Journals" (1991). These criteria are as follows:

> Each author should have participated sufficiently in the work to take public responsibility for the content. Authorship credit should be based only on substantial contributions to a) conception and design, or analysis and interpretation of data; and to b) drafting the article or revising it critically for important intellectual content; and on c) final approval of the version to be published. Conditions a), b), and c) must all be met.

With these criteria in mind, it would appear that Dr. Smith, who has had substantial input into the design and execution of the study and will help to prepare the manuscript, would be a valid coauthor, whereas Dr. Jones, who only provides clinic space, would not. On a practical level, and despite the guidelines offered, loose authorship is likely to be an ongoing problem given the incentives to publish and pressures to honor or please superiors. Some suggestions to address this problem are discussed in the conclusion of this chapter.

Disclosure of Financial Relationships

> A representative of a pharmaceutical firm contacts you and asks if you would be willing to give a talk on the treatment of a certain psychiatric disorder. You have received funds from this pharmaceutical firm to conduct research with this particular drug on this disorder and will be paid an honorarium for the presentation. Should you mention your relationship with the pharmaceutical firm at the talk? Should you indicate who is sponsoring your lecture at the time of the talk?

With the degree of industry-sponsored research in the current research climate, this is an important consideration. Accordingly, the Food and Drug Administration (FDA) is quite clear on this matter. The Draft Policy Statement on Industry-Supported Scientific and Educational Activities (1992) states the following (p. 3):

> Disclosure of Financial Relationships: The provider agrees to ensure meaningful disclosure at the time of the program, to the audience of a) the company's funding of the activity, and b) any significant relationship between the provider

and the company and between individual presenters or moderators and the company (e.g., employee, grant recipient, owner of significant interest or stock).

The publishers of medical journals have taken a similar stance on the disclosure issue (Kassirer and Angell 1993), so the answer in this case is clear: the financial relationship with the pharmaceutical company must be clearly stated at the time of the presentation. To the pharmaceutical industry's credit (and perhaps as evidence of its concerns about the FDA), most companies are generally rather forthright in reminding speakers of this obligation.

Subject Withdrawal From a Study

You are an investigator in an outpatient placebo-controlled trial of a new antidepressant medication: "Uplift." One of the patients in the study, Mr. Smith, who has been enrolled in the protocol for 3 weeks, seems to be deteriorating. The score on his Hamilton Rating Scale for Depression continues to go up, the patient reports difficulty sleeping, and he indicates that he has not been able to go to work for the last 3 days. His wife has contacted you by telephone to indicate that she is very concerned about him. What should you do?

All drug trials, especially those involving placebo controls, must have criteria in place to decide when subjects are to be removed from a study because of deterioration. In this case, it appears that the subject will need to be withdrawn from the study so that a clinically approved means of treating his depression can be instituted. The need for this subject to be dropped from the trial should be reported to the Institutional Review Board (IRB) at the time of annual renewal of the proposal, or if he deteriorates to the point at which he requires hospitalization, this should be reported immediately to both the sponsor and the IRB as a "serious adverse event."

Regulation of Clinical Research

You believe that an antidepressant medication may assist patients who have panic disorder. The antidepressant that you choose can be given in a variety of dosage forms. You are following two patients in the clinic who would be candidates for this study. You believe that it would be reasonable to give them the drug anyway, but your intent is to obtain information as "pilot data" and to publish the results. Does the IRB need to be involved?

This approach to treatment, especially when it involves the intent to seek publication and presumably involves the formal gathering of data, constitutes research and as such would need IRB approval. The distinction between practice and research is not always an easy one, particularly in a field in which so many therapeutic interventions that lack an FDA indication are used. From a practical standpoint (and probably in accord with the views of most IRBs), we believe that the gathering of data and the intent to publish constitute research. For a more thorough discussion of this topic, please refer to Levine (1986).

Selection of Data

After you begin a study, you find that you have treated two patients, but neither has responded. You decide to expand your sample and use a higher dose. To your encouragement, a dose double the original dose seems to be effective for the disorder in five additional patients. When you publish the results, should you mention the low-dose strategy that failed in the first two patients?

To omit mentioning the failure of the low-dose strategy would seem to come under Angell's rubric of selection of data. An important aspect of reporting scientific endeavors is to inform the reader fully of what was learned in the process. The IRB would of course have to be informed of these dosage changes *before* they were instituted (or, preferably, the protocol originally submitted might have anticipated the need for this).

Informed Consent

You are conducting an outpatient trial with the antidepressant "Uplift" to treat panic disorder. This drug is approved by the FDA for the treatment of depression but not panic. A potential patient for the study indicates that he very much wants to try this new drug and acknowledges that he has a 50% chance of receiving it because the trial is placebo-controlled, but he wants to find out whether he can get the drug outside of the protocol. Because the drug is not approved by the FDA for panic, you consider the possibility that you might not have to tell him about the availability of the drug for depression. Are you obligated to tell the patient about the availability of the drug outside of the protocol?

In this case, we return to the basic elements of informed consent. This entails not only stating the risks and benefits of being in a study but also informing potential subjects of the alternative treatments available. Given that most clinicians use drugs for non-FDA-approved indications frequently, it would seem to be a necessary part of the consent process to inform this subject of this alternative. To do otherwise would seem dishonest and potentially coercive.

> You are conducting a randomized outpatient trial of a new antidepressant: "Uplift." You receive notification from the manufacturer that several unexpected deaths have occurred secondary to hematological problems in patients receiving the medication and that no new patients should be started in the protocol. Are you obligated to notify the IRB of this change? Are you obligated to notify the patients already involved in the protocol?

This case again constitutes a consent issue. In 45 CFR 46.116b(5), "General Requirements for Informed Consent" stipulates inclusion of "a statement that significant new findings developed during the course of the research which may relate to the subject's willingness to continue participation will be provided to the subject." Because unexpected deaths in the course of a study do constitute "significant new findings," both the subjects already enrolled and the IRB will need to be notified promptly of this information. In the case of less obvious "adverse events," such as lesser medical complications or unexpected psychiatric events, it is advisable to notify the IRB and let it decide whether to notify subjects.

Duplication of Publication

> You are pursuing research with a rat model that shows great promise in suppressing binge eating, but you lack the sample size to provide adequate statistical power at this point. However, you are out of funds, your research assistant is starting graduate school at another university in a month, and you face an upcoming decision on tenure within the next year. Your mentor mentions that she is on the editorial board of a non-peer-reviewed journal that she believes would publish the paper. You are thinking that you could publish it now, and later, when the study has been completed after you obtain more funds and the data are complete, you could publish the paper in a prestigious journal too. What should you do?

This scenario involves the so-called Ingelfinger Rule, named after an editor of the *New England Journal of Medicine,* who in 1969 instituted a standard to protect the journal from publishing nonoriginal material (Angell and Kassirer 1991). This rule also was seen as a means to discourage public announcements of a scientific development before it undergoes the scrutiny of peer review and to minimize the practice of redundant publication. The rule holds that a manuscript will be considered for publication "only if its substance has not been submitted or reported elsewhere" (Angell and Kassirer 1991, p. 1372). Detractors have seen this as a means of holding up the announcement of important scientific findings, whereas others regard it as a mechanism to ensure meaningful scientific findings as well as the originality of the work to be published. Those submitting work to journals will find the Ingelfinger Rule almost universally invoked when they sign the declaration as to the originality of the published work. Therefore, in this scenario, the researcher would be best advised to wait until the work is finished.

Important exceptions to this rule are published abstracts or presentations at scientific meetings, although "we discourage authors from giving out more information, particularly figures and tables, than was presented at the meeting to their scientific peers" (Angell and Kassirer 1991, p. 1373). Accordingly, a reasonable alternative to publishing incomplete findings in a lesser journal is making a presentation on the preliminary results at a meeting or, lacking travel expenses, writing a letter to the editor discussing the preliminary nature of the results. Either way, it is hoped that progress in the research would be noted by the tenure committee.

As one can tell from the preceding discussion, the editors of journals are actively engaged in the problems of scientific misconduct. This is understandable, because they are at the receiving end of the publish-or-perish problem. Because of their roles, they have made many laudable efforts to clean up the process of writing, submitting, and publishing research data. Hence the seven stations in Angell (1983), the Ingelfinger Rule, and the call for more accountability in authorship.

Editors also have suggested rather ambitious systemwide reforms to ameliorate the pressure to publish or, as Maddox characterized it, weaken the "link between publication and personal success" (Maddox 1994, p. 353). Thomson (1994), discussing the issue in *American Scientist,* emphasized the need for authors to specify their contributions to a paper and longer grant periods to remove the pressure for quick results; he even suggested that under certain circumstances one's teaching commitment rather than the amount published might be evaluated. Angell (1986), in "Publish or Perish: A Proposal," suggested that "any institution or agency evaluating a researcher for promotion or for funding consider only, at most, the three articles the candidate considers to be his or her best in any given year, with a maximum of perhaps ten in any 5-year period" (p. 262). She maintains that this would improve the quality of medical research, lead to a situation in which "promotions and funding would more accurately reflect the quality of a researcher's work" and eliminate some of the "fluff in our huge scientific literature"

(p. 262). Whether a desirable outcome might accrue from such changes, the fact remains that researchers continue to publish as furiously as ever.

Conclusion and Some Thoughts About Remedies

Various regulatory agencies and the scientific community have invested much time in trying to come to grips with the problem of scientific misconduct. A persistent problem in the debate is how to define misconduct. There seems to be a consensus on what constitutes *fraud* (such as faking and falsifying data), but because of the legal burden of having to prove intent and injury in cases of fraud, the government has been trying to develop a definition of *misconduct* to streamline the process of prosecution (Schachman 1993, p. 148). In response to some rather notorious cases involving fabrication of data, the Public Health Service in the late 1980s proposed rules defining "misconduct in science" as "fabrication, falsification, plagiarism, deception or *other practices that seriously deviate from those that are commonly accepted within the scientific community* [italics added] for proposing, conducting or reporting research" (Schachman 1993). Cognizant of the dangers of an overly vague construct such as "deviation from commonly accepted norms," a 1992 panel convened by the National Academy of Sciences upheld the concept that fabrication, falsification, and plagiarism constituted misconduct. However, the panel went on to say that "misconduct in science does not include errors of judgment; errors in the recording, selection, or analysis of data; differences in opinion involving the interpretation of data; or misconduct unrelated to the research process" (Schachman 1993, p. 149).

In 1993, the U.S. Congress called for the creation of a 12-member panel of scientists, ethicists, and lawyers called the Commission on Research Integrity (CRI), which was given the mandate of identifying the weaknesses of the current system and providing recommendations to the DHHS. It was hoped that with the panel's recommendations, some of these issues might be resolved. However, the release of the CRI's report in November 1995 did little to quell the ongoing controversy about the definition of misconduct, and their other recommendations have come under significant criticism as well. The CRI's report suggested replacing the "seriously deviate from those that are commonly accepted within the scientific community" language with "misappropriation, interference and misrepresentation" as part of the definition of misconduct. However, critics charge that the definition is too vague and too broad (Wadman 1996), so the controversy continues.

There has also been significant resistance to the "whistle-blower's bill of rights" that the CRI recommended. A recent ORI survey documented a sizable number of whistle-blowers who experienced negative consequences ("Burdens of Proof of Misconduct" 1996). The legislation that created the CRI specifically called for protection of whistle-blowers, so it is anticipated that there will soon be action on the matter.

A 1994 "Opinion" piece in *Nature* ("What to Do About Scientific Misconduct" 1994) pointed out why agencies such as the ORI are having such difficulty in prosecuting cases such as Imanishi-Kari. The justice system is set up so that "any administrative decision by a federal agency will be open to appeal in the courts if it can be held that due process may have been denied" ("What to Do" 1994, p. 262). With these limitations and the federal judicial system in mind, the authors of the *Nature* editorial called for an increased accountability of the institutions where the investigators did the work (with monetary penalties if the institutions failed to police their researchers). Given these problems of federally mandating ethical behavior, this idea seems reasonable, and to the CRI's credit, this was one of its recommendations. As Kenneth Ryan, M.D., chair of the CRI, put it, "we want to have the government involved in felonies and to get institutions involved in misdemeanors" (Stone 1995, p. 449).

It would appear that institutional accountability of ethical behavior and the education of researchers in this area may become the standard as the debate over regulation of these issues unfolds. This appears to be a feasible way to handle this complex area as an alternative to overinvolvement of the federal government (which to date has proven unworkable). The CRI report did call for enhanced training in and support for conferences on research ethics at an institutional level, along with established procedures to deal with complaints. Although the cost of such programs has been a concern, these CRI recommendations have been better received than the controversial scientific misconduct definition and the whistle-blower protections. It is hoped that progress can be made toward establishing control of the issue within the purview of institutions rather than from the unwieldy and potentially restrictive mandates of the federal government.

CHAPTER 10

Writing Journal Articles

Learning to write articles for scientific journals is not an easy task, even for those who are good writers in general and who may have written many papers in college, medical school, or graduate school. Like most things, although this task often seems enormous at first, it becomes easier with time. The best way to learn to write journal articles is simply to do it and learn from experience and feedback from others (colleagues, reviewers, editors) throughout the process.

It has been said that scientific papers should already be written before the data are collected. This statement has some truth; the literature review, methodology, and, to some extent, the discussion should be in draft form before the experiment is actually completed, assuming that the manuscript describes hypothesis-driven research. However, considerable time often passes between the design of an experiment and its completion; thus, the researcher must re-review the literature in detail before completing a final draft of the manuscript to ensure that the introduction, discussion, and references are up to date. Also, it is important to bear in mind that published papers represent work that was done at least 6 months to 2 years before publication, and the most recent references can be better obtained by attending meetings or requesting preprints from others who are working in the field. This strategy obviously becomes easier as a researcher becomes more advanced in a field and places junior investigators at a disadvantage. Nonetheless, the most recent work in a field is found by talking to the people doing the cutting-edge work and then trying to incorporate reference to this work into the manuscript.

Getting Started

Once an investigator has data to write up, where does he or she begin?

Writing a rough draft is the first step. Dictation or word processing can be used (some think better when they are not typing, whereas others think better when they can actually see what they are writing), but the draft must be done, even though it probably will have shortcomings and will need extensive reworking. For many, completing this first draft is getting over the hump, and most junior investigators find that the process becomes easier after writing the first draft.

Scientific writing should be direct and concise. Long, complicated sentence structure should be avoided. The writing must be clear to understand what the investigator is saying. Hemingway probably would have been a good scientific writer. Although it may be tempting at times to be a Faulkner, complex sentences usually have no place in scientific journals. When in doubt, cut and simplify is the rule.

Reworking the Manuscript

The researcher also must stick to the data and write conservatively. Use of speculation must be made clear. The writer generally has more free rein in book chapters, but regardless of the type of manuscript, the difference between data-based interpretations and speculation must be clear. The writer has to be careful to use certain words appropriately: *significant* in a scientific article is meant to imply statistical significance; *trend, different, increasing* and *decreasing,* and *greater* or *lesser* all will be assumed to suggest statistical concepts, not descriptions. These words should not be used to imply another meaning unless they are so defined.

Deciding early in the preparation process where the paper will be submitted for publication is also useful because the requirements and styles of journals vary. Reviewing several articles from the journal in which one hopes to publish is a way to determine the appropriate style and length of the paper.

Some beginning writers occasionally make the mistake of being overly critical of the work of others. They may attempt to establish the importance of their own work by subtly, and sometimes more overtly, downgrading earlier work that has been done in the field, focusing primarily on the weaknesses of earlier studies. This is unwise. First, research builds on the work of others, and it is unjust to judge work that was done at an earlier point in the development of a field by contemporary standards. Second, from a practical standpoint, the people being criticized often are the reviewers of new manuscripts, and researchers who wish to continue to work in a particular field should establish good professional relationships with them. Therefore, investigators should view themselves and their work as standing on the shoulders of others, and they should not attempt to make their own work important by degrading the work of others. This does not mean that judicial criticism is inappropriate; indeed, it is necessary to be appropriately critical in the review of the studies preceding one's work, but one should attempt to be even-handed and impersonal. When in doubt, the investigator should be generous and always strive for balance.

Problems and Pitfalls

Plagiarism, a process that can creep in unknowingly during a literature review, must be avoided. Some investigators take notes while reading articles and later use these notes to dictate or type the literature review. In this process, verbatim material may be inadvertently incorporated. If this is done, it is extremely important to cite the work of others. This is also a problem when people write a series of articles on the same or similar topics. A researcher often may plagiarize his or her own work by using the same phrases or lines again. The writer must try to be aware of this and to remember to amend or rewrite those passages that seem all too familiar.

If the statistical write-up in the paper is complex and sophisticated, a statistical consultant should review it and make suggestions, unless the researcher is well versed in the area of statistics.

Several additional problems must be avoided in writing articles. One we have mentioned that deserves emphasis is overinterpretation. Investigators may overinterpret the importance of their findings in the enthusiasm for their own work. They want readers to share their excitement and to be impressed by the results of all of their labors. Unfortunately, when writing up results, one must try to set aside such personal issues and view the data dispassionately, as when one is reviewing the data of others. As has often been said, it is important to stick to the data. By extension, many investigators find it difficult to discern and adequately discuss the shortcomings and limitations of their own work. There is no such thing as a perfect study. One thing that researchers should try to learn from each experiment is how it could have been done better. Therefore, the writer should think like a reviewer or a reader and, in a prominent place in the discussion section, carefully review the limitations of the work and possible ways to address these limitations in future research.

Authors commonly confuse the introduction and the discussion, letting discussion material filter into the introduction. The introduction should be a brief overview that includes the necessary literature and ideas but avoids an in-depth discussion of the results of or the importance of the study. In contrast, the discussion can be more expansive and discursive. The in-depth literature review belongs in the discussion, and the literature should be tied to the results.

Another point of concern in discussing the implications of one's results is sample size. Reviews have shown that many of the questions asked in most published studies have used study samples that result in a power that is inadequate to answer such questions. Reviewers increasingly point out this problem. The investigator must adequately assess and discuss whether the sample size was adequate to answer the questions that were posed and, if not, suggest ways in which this can be addressed in future research.

Choosing a Journal

In thinking about where to submit a paper for publication, several issues must be considered. First, the researcher should ask, "How important is this study, and what readership would be interested in it?" If the study is so important that it should be of interest to many groups of scientists (a rare situation), the results may be publishable in the most widely read journals, such as *Science* or *Nature*. If the study is of importance to many medical researchers, but probably not other scientific readers, it is at a different level and appropriate for a leading medical journal. Such a manuscript might merit publication in a major medical journal read by practitioners around the world, such as the *New England Journal of Medicine*, the *Journal of the American Medical Association*, or *Lancet*.

Most of the clinical psychiatric literature does not justify either of these levels of exposure and, instead, if considered of general importance to the field, should be directed to one of the major psychiatric journals (i.e., *American Journal of Psychiatry*, *Archives of General Psychiatry*, *British Journal of Psychiatry*, and *Biological Psychiatry*) or to more subspecialized journals, depending on the nature of the material (e.g., *Journal of Affective Disorders*, *Psychosomatic Medicine*, *Journal of Clinical Psychopharmacology*, and *International Journal of Eating Disorders*). Also, some additional psychiatric journals (e.g., *Journal of Clinical Psychiatry*, *Journal of Nervous and Mental Disease*, and *Comprehensive*

Psychiatry) publish articles on general psychiatric issues, usually including papers that are not at a level of importance meriting placement in a major journal such as the *American Journal of Psychiatry* but are of interest nonetheless.

The author must be realistic about these issues. Sending an article to a journal when there is little or no chance of the journal accepting it may take a great deal of time and may delay publication of the article until its importance to the field is diminished. Again, advice from others can be very helpful here.

In preparing a journal article, it is important to follow the instructions to authors for that particular journal, which vary dramatically among the different psychiatric journals. (This step has become less a problem with word-processing software that reformats references automatically into any of various journal styles.) The psychological journals have a more a uniform system (*Publication Manual of the American Psychological Association*) than the psychiatric journals.

One good way to decide which journal is appropriate for an article is to look at its reference list. This shows where other articles in this field are being published. Also, it is sometimes helpful to call the editor of the potential target journal, particularly if a review article is planned, to find out whether he or she might be interested in a particular work.

Authorship and Data Ownership

Authorship of articles has become a problem in all scientific fields, because the number of authors for articles generally has been increasing as research becomes more complex and as the "publish or perish" mentality leads researchers in the direction of overinclusion (Thomson 1994). Various journals have suggested different solutions, and the topic will likely remain an ongoing source of debate.

Another issue concerns data ownership. Universities in different states have handled this in various ways. For example, some universities have ruled that the investigator owns the data he or she produces, but elsewhere, the university at which the work is performed owns the data. Investigators must be aware of the rules and regulations at their particular institution.

Polishing the Manuscript

Feedback from others is essential. After the second or third draft, others should read the paper. It is often useful to have a layperson, such as a significant other who is not in the field, read the article. If he or she cannot follow it (aside from the technical aspects), something is probably wrong with the way it is written.

The other authors should be involved in the process of manuscript preparation from the beginning and must sign off on the final draft; the first author should carefully read and/or listen to their comments at each stage. Outside researchers not involved with the work also should read the paper. Researchers can all learn to be better writers, and it is important not to be easily offended but to be open to others' suggestions.

Editorial Decisions

"Not Accepted But Will Reconsider With Revisions"

A journal may not accept a manuscript but is willing to reconsider that decision if the author makes the proper revisions. The letter sent by the journal's editor often sounds more negative than it really is. At this point, the author should review the suggestions carefully and respond to each, because these will generally strengthen the article (and because the original reviewers often will see the revised manuscript again). The following are some rules of thumb:

1. If the author does not want to make a change (or changes) that is suggested, he or she should defend why this decision was made in the cover letter back to the editor.

2. The author should not become hostile or defensive.

3. The author should attempt to learn from these reviews. This is free feedback from other researchers in the field. By studying this feedback, the author can learn much about improving their writing, organizing and presenting data, and methods of conducting experiments.

4. The author should return the manuscript while it is still fresh in the reviewers' and the editor's minds. An author may have lost interest in the work at this point and may not want to polish a manuscript further, but he or she should not delay. Returning the manuscript quickly shows that the author continues to be interested in the work and the journal and prevents the manuscript from becoming out of date.

Rejected

Rejection of a manuscript is usually difficult to take. Most authors who receive a rejection letter (and all do) usually are tempted to put the manuscript and the reviewers' comments in a bottom drawer and try to ignore them for a while.

Reviewers' comments can be hurtful. The best reviewers, and the most useful reviews, are nonhostile but helpful and supportive. Beginning reviewers sometimes are more likely to say potentially hurtful things in their reviews in an effort to seem knowledgeable and critical. Nonetheless, authors can learn a great deal from a good review. A good reviewer can teach the author much about the strengths and weaknesses of his or her writing style and can point out any idiosyncrasies that the author may wish to correct in future manuscripts. Reviewers can help their colleagues with suggestions, which benefits the entire field.

Accepted

Unfortunately, when a manuscript is accepted, the job still is not over. First, the delay between acceptance and actual publication may be long enough that parts of a manuscript, especially the literature review, may have to be augmented or even rewritten when the work comes back in galley proof form. Journals are generally reluctant to allow the author to do much of this, but changes in the field may have been important enough that parts of a manuscript have to be rewritten. When this issue is questionable, the author should discuss it with the editor or editorial assistant at the journal, particularly if the changes are substantial.

The author also should review the galley proofs to determine what changes the copyeditors have made to the manuscript. They may have introduced errors, which can be noted, but more commonly, they will have significantly improved on the writing style. Again, comparing the original submission with the galley proofs will allow the author to see the elements of writing that may need modification in future work.

Conclusion

Like most academic tasks, writing journal articles is a skill that is developed over time. Authors must be open to the suggestions of others (colleagues, reviewers, editors), thick-skinned, and, above all, prompt. Becoming a productive clinical researcher requires one to publish, so he or she must jump in, write up the results, submit the manuscripts, promptly return the revised manuscript, resubmit rejected manuscripts, and learn throughout the process.

CHAPTER 11

Reviewing Journal Articles

Reviewing journal articles is a topic about which little has been written and is rarely, if ever, systematically taught, even in an informal manner. Instead, it is a generally unstandardized task that one learns haphazardly by trial and error. It is unfortunate that this somewhat intuitive task plays such a significant role in the lives of many academicians.

The Objective

When potential reviewers receive a request from a journal editor to review a manuscript, they must understand what they are being asked to do. An editor, or associate editor, who may know very little about the topic of the paper, must decide whether the paper in question should be published in his or her journal. To make an informed decision, editors often need help in the form of outside reviewers. The journal may have a formal editorial board to which an editor can turn for consultation, or he or she may rely on a more informal network of colleagues. The editorial decision requires a careful and thoughtful examination of the paper in terms of its scientific merit, methodology, clarity of writing, thoroughness of the literature review, and soundness in conclusion. Here, reviewers should not expound on their own personal ideas or theories but should instead provide an evenhanded commentary on the merits of the work that will ultimately help the editor make a decision about its suitability for publication.

The Request

When a reviewer receives a request to review a manuscript, he or she must consider a couple of issues. First, is he or she familiar enough with the topic to provide a review? The editor has sent it to the reviewer because he or she believes that the reviewer does know the topic, but sometimes this is not the case. For example, the overall topic of the manuscript may seem appropriate, but the focus is on a methodology or population outside of the reviewer's expertise. If this happens, the reviewer should feel free to return the manuscript to the editor with a simple explanation that it is outside of his or her area of expertise. The reviewer may wish to offer names of individuals who would provide a competent review of the paper.

Second, can the reviewer meet the deadline that the editor is requesting? It is frustrating for editors and authors to wait for lengthy periods to receive the reviewer's comment, and such delays slow the whole process of the dissemination of science. Most editors are generous in allowing 4–6 weeks for a review. However, if the reviewer does not think that he or she could do the review within that interval, for whatever reason, he or she should let the editor know that he or she simply does not have the time. Some reviewers, early in their careers, fear that they will never be asked to review a manuscript if they turn one down, and this could be professionally damaging. Being tardy in one's review is far more likely to suggest to the editor that the reviewer should be passed over next time. Reviewers who let the editor know, when returning the manuscript, that they are willing to review articles in the future are likely to receive more requests.

Reading the Manuscript

When reading a manuscript for a review, it helps to have a slightly different frame of reference from that used when reading papers for other reasons. Specifically, it seems best to read the paper while keeping in mind the following questions:

- What additions would make this paper better?
- What are the weaknesses?
- What does not make sense?
- What is missing?

The reviewer should remember that no paper is perfect, and this is an opportunity to enhance the quality of a paper that may eventually reach the scientific literature. In this sense, the reviewer becomes a contributor (although unrecognized) to the work. Furthermore, such a supportive and collegial approach to conducting the review not only enhances the quality of the scientific literature but also is appreciated by the editor and the author.

Writing the Comments to Authors

The central task of the reviewer is to compose a statement that embodies his or her opinion on the positive and negative aspects of the paper he or she is reviewing. This information is critical to the review because that part of the review is actually returned to the author to improve the paper. Usually, comments to authors are 1–3 pages. Writing a single paragraph or two is likely to be of limited benefit to the editor and the authors. Furthermore, general nonspecific comments to the authors also are minimally useful. The reviewer should be as thorough in the written review as in his or her own reading.

The review itself should be concise and anchored to specific identified features of the paper. One approach is to construct the comments to the authors in the same format as the manuscript itself. For example, the review comments would be organized in the following order: "Introduction," "Method," "Results," and "Discussion," with more specific detailed comments at the end (e.g., comments on spelling, grammar, typographical errors). The following sections include a few ideas about useful feedback in each of these categories.

Introduction

The reviewer may benefit from asking two questions about the "Introduction":

1. Is it comprehensive in its coverage of the appropriate literature? If not, the reviewer should point this out and might provide a few citations that the authors could include.

2. Have the authors provided a reasonable conceptual or theoretical framework that allows the reader to understand what they were testing or examining in the study? Usually, the final paragraph in the "Introduction" lays out theoretical hypotheses that were tested in the study and are later discussed in the "Results" section. Any concerns the reviewer has about

the clarity of the hypotheses or their theoretical accuracy should be mentioned in this section of the commentary.

Methods

In the "Methods" section, the reviewer's comments will likely become much more specific. Anything that the reviewer finds concerning or laudable about the methodology and research design used in the study should be mentioned in this section. Was the sample adequate? Were subjects ascertained in an appropriate manner? Are there potential confounds between the groups that have not been addressed in the paper? Were the measures adequate, and did the authors provide a reasonable description of their psychometric properties with appropriate citations? Did the authors describe the procedures adequately, particularly in complex laboratory studies in which subjects undergo an elaborate protocol? Is the design clear, and have the authors adequately described their approach to the data analysis that is presented in the "Results" section?

These and other questions may cross the reviewer's mind as he or she reads the "Methods" section. Whenever possible, the reviewer may offer suggestions about how authors may overcome problems that have been identified. This is helpful because it again facilitates a process by which the paper will be improved rather than being a highly critical and belittling experience in which the author's methods are criticized without constructive comment.

Results

In the "Results" section, the reviewer should consider several general issues:

1. Was the statistical analysis of the data appropriate? Even if it was appropriate, could another analysis or additional analyses enhance the overall examination of the data? If the reviewer does not believe that the analysis was appropriate, he or she should clearly state why and offer alternatives.

2. Have the authors presented the findings of the study in a clear and straightforward manner?

3. Is descriptive information missing (e.g., means, standard deviations, standard errors, or percentages) that is necessary to understand the results?

4. Are the tables and figures relevant? A reviewer can be very helpful to the authors in the examination of tables and figures. Has the author used the table or the figure to depict a critical portion of the results? Are the data

understandable in the format used, or are there better alternatives? Can tables or figure be deleted?

5. Have the authors applied and interpreted the statistical analyses appropriately? This should not be confused with the authors' attempts to explain or interpret the meanings of the findings but instead refers only to the authors' completion and interpretation of the data analysis. In this portion of the review, the reviewer can comment on many specific issues regarding the statistics, such as statistical power, alpha levels, appropriateness of particular statistical models, and selection of error terms.

Discussion

A good discussion should be the authors' best effort to explain the significant findings in the study and relate them to the available literature. Here, the authors essentially are allowed to expound on how they account for what they have found. Reviewers can help by posing alternative explanations for the findings or by pointing out what they believe is lacking in the authors' explanation. The reviewer can point out other works in the field or make references to certain theories that may help the authors to broaden the discussion of their findings.

When the methodology or statistical analysis is considered to be inappropriate or problematic, the reviewer will have problems with the "Discussion." He or she may have very little to say about the "Discussion" because the results themselves are thought to be problematic. Usually a reviewer can simply indicate that he or she had difficulty commenting on the "Discussion" because of the previously mentioned concerns about the methods and/or statistics. He or she may note that if these concerns are addressed satisfactorily, then he or she can comment more appropriately on the "Discussion."

Typically, in the "Discussion," authors will offer disclaimers about the limitations of their study or recommendations for future studies. In his or her consideration of the "Discussion" section, the reviewer can offer additional helpful ideas about these topics. For example, what would be a reasonable follow-up to this study? How should the results of the present study inform and influence future studies?

References

Usually, reviewers do not check each reference in great detail. That is, they do not ensure that each reference cited in the text of the manuscript is included in the reference list or that each reference included in the reference list is cited in the text. However, problems like this, or other types of problems (e.g., incomplete information) can simply be pointed out to the authors at the end of the comments to the authors.

Information for the Editor

In addition to providing detailed comments to the author, reviewers also are generally asked to complete a form that is used only by the editor and is not shared with the author. On such a form, reviewers are typically asked to rate the manuscript along several dimensions, such as likely interest to the readership of the journal, importance of the study, coverage of the literature, methodological quality of the study, clarity of presentation, and theoretical grounding. Also, reviewers are asked to recommend whether the paper should be published; they can suggest that the paper be 1) accepted as it is, 2) revised and resubmitted, 3) most likely declined because of the need for major revisions, or 4) rejected. The information from all of the reviewers is integrated by the editor, who makes the ultimate decision about the status of the paper.

Summary

Reviewing journal articles is an important task that is a critical contribution to the scientific research community but is often unrecognized. However, without good journal article reviewers, the information that is published in journals could be severely compromised. A strong critical review that identifies clearly the strengths and weaknesses of a paper, along with recommendations for improvement, is important. Journal article reviews should not be opportunities to yield hostile attacks on colleagues' work, and every effort should be made to provide constructive criticism of ideas and methods. Such a thorough but positive and constructive approach to journal article reviewing will benefit individual authors, editors, and possibly the reviewer when he or she submits a paper for editorial review.

CHAPTER 12

Scientific Presentations

The practice or art of orally and visually presenting scientific material is a central feature of a research career. Despite this, most researchers never receive any training in this area. Over time, they learn to improve their presentations through trial and error, often by observing effective presentations by colleagues. Frequently, researchers will make a scientific presentation as a preliminary step to preparing a scientific paper. That is, when they have preliminary information from a study, they may submit an abstract to a professional meeting as an oral presentation and then receive feedback, which they hope will enhance the quality of their written manuscript. Professional meetings typically devote large blocks of time to oral scientific presentations; both junior and senior researchers have an opportunity to communicate with others about their studies and gain feedback about their research effort. Also, lengthy delays in publication often can be avoided in presentations because the data presented can be updated to include the more recent results.

Types of Scientific Presentations

Oral Presentation

The first type of scientific presentation we discuss is the oral report or oral presentation. Oral paper sessions generally have a standard structure at most professional meetings in psychiatry and psychology. A group of six or more papers is presented in a 75- to 90-minute period. Generally, each presenter provides an overview of a single study that was conducted, including an introduction, methods, results, and a discussion. Typically, someone is designated to preside over the paper session, and each speaker is asked to present for approximately 10–12 minutes, with an additional 3–5 minutes for questions and discussion from the audience. The oral presentation is usually accompanied by slides or overhead projector transparencies that summarize important information in the oral presentation. Generally, it is wise not to have more than 1 or 2 slides per minute in an oral presentation. In other words, the standard 10- to 12-minute talk should have no more than 20–25 slides shown during the presentation and often has fewer.

Symposium

A second format for presentations is the symposium, a series of oral presentations with related content that provide a more extensive examination of a single topic than the typical oral paper session. At most large professional meetings, the symposium chairperson organizes the symposium; typically, he or she contacts individual speakers at the time that abstracts for the meeting are being submitted and invites them to submit a proposal for the symposium, which the chairperson submits to the conference organizers. The chairperson is responsible for coordinating the topics to be covered in the symposium. For the individual speaker in the symposium, the presentation is fundamentally the same as that in an oral presentation. A standard amount of time is allotted to each speaker, and a discussant usually appears at the end of the symposium—a person (sometime the symposium chairperson) who provides integrative comments on the various talks. Again, these oral presentations are often accompanied by slides or overhead transparencies.

Poster Session

A third format for scientific presentations is the poster session. A favorite avenue of junior investigators to gain experience in scientific presentations, poster sessions are usually allotted substantial amounts of time at scientific meetings. Similar to the oral presentation, the poster session is generally a presentation of a single research study. The entire study, however, is presented on a large (i.e., usually 4 × 6 feet) poster. The poster generally has sections for the introduction, background, methods, results, discussion, and references. The poster presenter typically stands next to the poster during the session and is available for discussion during the entire poster presentation session, which can be 1–3 hours. Also, many poster presenters will provide interested individuals with a written summary of their presentation. Typically, during a poster session, a large number of posters are being presented, resulting in a relaxed, informal atmosphere in which researchers can discuss studies with presenters in an unstructured manner. This is an excellent opportunity for young investigators to present their data to colleagues in a generally supportive and nonthreatening format.

Invited Address

Another distinctive format for scientific presentations is the colloquium, or grand rounds, or some other form of an invited address. These presentations are lengthier than the previously discussed presentations, and the presenter may discuss more than one study in detail or provide a review and survey of studies in a particular area of scientific work. Typically, such presentations are made in psychiatry or psychology departments within medical schools or colleges of arts and science. The department may have a designated weekly scientific presentation in which its own faculty and others are invited to give talks. This type of presentation is very different from the standard oral presentation and requires considerably more organization to effectively weave multiple studies into one coherent talk that will last approximately 40–70 minutes, depending on the format. Generally, more experienced presenters or researchers are invited to give such lectures.

Preparing for the Standard Oral Presentation

Once an abstract proposal has been accepted for presentation at a scientific meeting, the clinician must think about how to present the study in the amount of time allotted (e.g., 10 minutes). Without question, the single biggest problem that arises in oral presentations is that the presenter runs out of time before presenting all the intended material. In this unfortunate and uncomfortable situation, the individual presiding over the session may be fervently trying, with various notes and nonverbal gestures, to get the speaker to stop talking, while the speaker realizes that he or she has to cut the talk but is not sure how to do so, and while the remaining speakers are becoming concerned that their own time will now be cut short. The following suggestions may help to prevent this dilemma:

1. *Outline the talk.* The presenter should outline the talk, highlighting only the most essential points. The best oral presentations do not provide ex-

haustive detailed reviews of the literature, do not go into exquisite detail about various measures and their psychometric properties, and do not give elaborate descriptions of statistical procedures. The presenter should speak telegraphically and clearly state the essential points.

2. *Open strong.* The talk should be started in a manner that will gain the audience's attention. The introduction is essential and will "set the stage," if done well.

3. *Accentuate key points.* Slides should accentuate key points and summarize significant material. For example, the presenter might want to show a slide that lists several studies that he or she has reviewed in preparation for the talk. Each study should not be reviewed, but the audience should simply be referred to the slide while the speaker summarizes the major points that have been abstracted.

4. *Get to the "Results" section quickly.* The audience wants to hear about the results of the study being presented. Therefore, the speaker should not spend any more time than needed reviewing literature and presenting methods.

5. *Use handouts.* A handout with results in tabular or figure format is very useful. The presenter should provide an address where the audience members can write to him or her about the talk.

6. *Leave time for questions.* The presenter should leave time for two or three questions, which should be answered in a nondefensive, straightforward manner. If he or she does not know the answer, he or she should say so.

Audiovisual Material

Slides are an extremely important facet of a good scientific presentation. They allow data to be summarized succinctly and clearly. However, another major problem that can plague a scientific presentation is a series of slides that are unreadable to the audience. We suggest the following basic guidelines:

1. The amount of information contained in a single slide should be limited to two or three main points. These points should be placed in the center portion of the slide, and the slide should not be filled with words or numbers.

2. If possible, data should be presented in figures that are amenable to visual interpretation, such as bar graphs, pie charts, and line graphs. Large tables of numbers should be avoided if possible. If a table with numbers

must be used, a hard copy of the table should be given to members of the audience to examine.

3. When creating the slides, the clinician should think carefully about the size of the letters and the color of the slides. Letters and numbers should be large enough to be read with the naked eye without projection. It is best, if possible, to have the slides presented in a single color combination. Printed slides can be made in numerous color combinations. Black on white is easy to read but may be too bright for the audience. Blue, green, and red on white may glare and be difficult to read. White on blue is readable in half-light and is quite easy on the viewer's eyes. New computer programs allow various combinations to be tested. These programs are particularly helpful in terms of using colors to accent major points to the audience. Sufficient contrast between colors is necessary to read the slide.

4. The presenter should practice the talk before the presentation; he or she should use a clock or a watch if the time will be limited. If the talk cannot consistently be completed within the limited amount of time, it must be cut. Slides also should be reviewed before the presentation. There is nothing worse than arriving at a destination far from home with slides that have not been reviewed and discovering that the slide has an error or that one slide is missing. Many conferences have a preparation room in which slides can be reviewed in the building where the talk will be given. Reviewing the slides here is a useful way to ensure that all of the slides are in order and offers a final opportunity to review the talk.

5. The presenter should be familiar with the use of a pointer. A speaker who stands at a podium and runs across a stage to point at particular details in a slide can be very distracting. Typically, a wooden pointer or a laser pointer will be available to the speaker, and effective use of the pointer can enhance the quality of the presentation.

Summary

The scientific presentation is an important part of any researcher's career and an important aspect of the scientific process. Well-organized, well-planned, and succinct talks will be the most satisfying to the audience and will permit the presenter to leave the venue feeling that she or he has effectively communicated his or her ideas. The researcher must remember that he or she is trying to communicate extremely complex information to an audience who has never heard about the study previously. If the audience did not understand the talk, the major objective has been missed, even if the speaker thought that it went well.

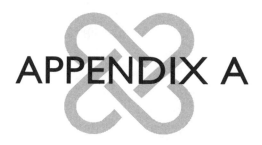

APPENDIX A

The Nuremberg Code

1. The voluntary consent of the human subject is absolutely essential.

   This means that the person involved should have legal capacity to give consent; should be so situated as to be able to exercise free power of choice, without the intervention of any element of force, fraud, deceit, duress, overreaching, or other ulterior form of constraint or coercion; and should have sufficient knowledge and comprehension of the elements of the subject matter involved as to enable him to make an understanding and enlightened decision.

   This latter element requires that before the acceptance of an affirmative decision by the experimental subject there should be made known to him the nature, duration, and purpose of the experiment; the method and means by which it is to be conducted; all inconveniences and hazards reasonably to be expected; and the effects upon his health or person which may possibly come from his participation in the experiment.

   The duty and responsibility for ascertaining the quality of the consent rests upon each individual who initiates, directs or engages in the experiment. It is a personal duty and responsibility which may not be delegated to another with impunity.

From *Trials of War Criminals Before the Nuremberg Military Tribunals Under Control Council Law No. 10, Vol. 2, Nuremberg, October 1946–April 1949.* Washington, DC, U.S. Government Printing Office, 1949, pp. 181–182.

2. The experiment should be such as to yield fruitful results for the good of society, unprocurable by other methods or means of study, and not random and unnecessary in nature.

3. The experiment should be so designed and based on the results of animal experimentation and a knowledge of the natural history of the disease or other problem under study that the anticipated results will justify the performance of the experiment.

4. The experiment should be so conducted as to avoid all unnecessary physical and mental suffering and injury.

5. No experiment should be conducted where there is an a priori reason to believe that death or disabling injury will occur; except perhaps, in those experiments where the experimental physicians also serve as subjects.

6. The degree of risk to be taken should never exceed that determined by the humanitarian importance of the problem to be solved by the experiment.

7. Proper preparations should be made and adequate facilities provided to protect the experimental subject against even remote possibilities of injury, disability, or death.

8. The experiment should be conducted only by scientifically qualified persons. The highest degree of skill and care should be required through all stages of the experiment of those who conduct or engage in the experiment.

9. During the course of the experiment the human subject should be at liberty to bring the experiment to an end if he has reached the physical or mental state where continuation of the experiment seems to him to be impossible.

10. During the course of the experiment the scientist in charge must be prepared to terminate the experiment at any stage, if he has probable cause to believe, in the exercise of the good faith, superior skill, and careful judgment required of him, that a continuation of the experiment is likely to result in injury, disability, or death to the experimental subject.

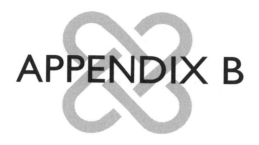

APPENDIX B

World Medical Association Declaration of Helsinki

World Medical Association Declaration of Helsinki: Recommendations Guiding Physicians in Biomedical Research Involving Human Subjects

Introduction

It is the mission of the physician to safeguard the health of the people. His or her knowledge and conscience are dedicated to the fulfillment of this mission.

The Declaration of Geneva of the World Medical Association binds the physician with the words, "The health of my patient will be my first consideration," and the International Code of Medical Ethics declares that, "A physi-

Adopted by the 18th World Medical Assembly, Helsinki, Finland, 1964, and amended by the 29th World Medical Assembly, Tokyo, Japan, 1975; 35th World Medical Assembly, Venice, Italy, 1983; 41st World Medical Assembly, Hong Kong, 1989; and the 48th General Assembly, Somerset West, Republic of South Africa, 1996.

Reprinted from *Protecting Human Research Subjects: Institutional Review Board Guidebook,* Appendix B. Office of Protection from Research Risks. Washington, DC, U.S. Government Printing Office, 1993.

cian shall act only in the patient's interest when providing medical care which might have the effect of weakening the physical and mental condition of the patient."

The purpose of biomedical research involving human subjects must be to improve diagnostic, therapeutic and prophylactic procedures and the understanding of the etiology and pathogenesis of disease.

In current medical practice most diagnostic, therapeutic or prophylactic procedures involve hazards. This applies especially to biomedical research.

Medical progress is based on research which ultimately must rest in part on experimentation involving human subjects.

In the field of biomedical research a fundamental distinction must be recognized between medical research in which the aim is essentially diagnostic or therapeutic for a patient, and medical research, the essential object of which is purely scientific and without implying direct diagnostic or therapeutic value to the person subjected to the research.

Special caution must be exercised in the conduct of research which may affect the environment, and the welfare of animals used for research must be respected.

Because it is essential that the results of laboratory experiments be applied to human beings to further scientific knowledge and to help suffering humanity, the World Medical Association has prepared the following recommendations as a guide to every physician in biomedical research involving human subjects. They should be kept under review in the future. It must be stressed that the standards as drafted are only a guide to physicians all over the world. Physicians are not relieved from criminal, civil and ethical responsibilities under the laws of their own countries.

I. Basic Principles

1. Biomedical research involving human subjects must conform to generally accepted scientific principles and should be based on adequately performed laboratory and animal experimentation and on a thorough knowledge of the scientific literature.

2. The design and performance of each experimental procedure involving human subjects should be clearly formulated in an experimental protocol which should be transmitted for consideration, comment and guidance to a specially appointed committee independent of the investigator and the sponsor provided that this independent committee is in confor-

mity with the laws and regulations of the country in which the research experiment is performed.

3. Biomedical research involving human subjects should be conducted only by scientifically qualified persons and under the supervision of a clinically competent medical person. The responsibility for the human subject must always rest with a medically qualified person and never rest on the subject of the research, even though the subject has given his or her consent.

4. Biomedical research involving human subjects cannot legitimately be carried out unless the importance of the objective is in proportion to the inherent risk to the subject.

5. Every biomedical research project involving human subjects should be preceded by careful assessment of predictable risks in comparison with foreseeable benefits to the subject or to others. Concern for the interests of the subject must always prevail over the interests of science and society.

6. The right of the research subject to safeguard his or her integrity must always be respected. Every precaution should be taken to respect the privacy of the subject and to minimize the impact of the study on the subject's physical and mental integrity and on the personality of the subject.

7. Physicians should abstain from engaging in research projects involving human subjects unless they are satisfied that the hazards involved are believed to be predictable. Physicians should cease any investigation if the hazards are found to outweigh the potential benefits.

8. In publication of the results of his or her research, the physician is obliged to preserve the accuracy of the results. Reports of experimentation not in accordance with the principles laid down in the Declaration should not be accepted for publication.

9. In any research on human beings, each potential subject must be adequately informed of the aims, methods, anticipated benefits and potential hazards of the study and the discomfort it may entail. He or she should be informed that he or she is at liberty to abstain from participation in the study and that he or she is free to withdraw his or her consent to participation at any time. The physician should then obtain the subject's freely given informed consent, preferably in writing.

10. When obtaining informed consent for the research project the physician should be particularly cautious if the subject is in a dependent relationship to him or her or may consent under duress. In that case the informed con-

sent should be obtained by a physician who is not engaged in the investigation and who is completely independent of this official relationship.

11. In case of legal incompetence, informed consent should be obtained from the legal guardian in accordance with national legislation. Where physical or mental incapacity makes it impossible to obtain informed consent, or when the subject is a minor, permission from the responsible relative replaces that of the subject in accordance with national legislation. Whenever the minor child is in fact able to give a consent, the minor's consent must be obtained in addition to the consent of the minor's legal guardian.

12. The research protocol should always contain a statement of the ethical considerations involved and should indicate that the principles enunciated in the present Declaration are complied with.

II. Medical Research Combined With Clinical Care (Clinical Research)

1. In the treatment of the sick person, the physician must be free to use a new diagnostic and therapeutic measure, if in his or her judgment it offers hope of saving life, reestablishing health or alleviating suffering.

2. The potential benefits, hazards and discomfort of a new method should be weighted against the advantages of the best current diagnostic and therapeutic methods.

3. In any medical study, every patient—including those of a control group, if any—should be assured of the best proven diagnostic and therapeutic method. This does not exclude the use of inert placebo in studies where no proven diagnostic or therapeutic method exists.

4. The refusal of the patient to participate in a study must never interfere with the physician-patient relationship.

5. If the physician considers it essential not to obtain informed consent, the specific reasons for this proposal should be stated in the experimental protocol for transmission to the independent committee.

6. The physician can combine medical research with professional care, the objective being the acquisition of new medical knowledge, only to the extent that medical research is justified by its potential diagnostic or therapeutic value for the patient.

III. Nontherapeutic Biomedical Research Involving Human Subjects (Non-Clinical Biomedical Research)

1. In the purely scientific application of medical research carried out on a human being, it is the duty of the physician to remain the protector of life and health of that person on whom biomedical research is being carried out.

2. The subjects should be volunteers—either healthy persons or patients for whom the experimental design is not related to the patient's illness.

3. The investigator or the investigating team should discontinue the research if in his/her or their judgment it may, if continued, be harmful to the individual.

4. In research on man, the interest of science and society should never take precedence over considerations related to the well-being of the subject.

APPENDIX C

Research Involving the U.S. Food and Drug Administration

In this appendix we summarize what is involved in doing experimental drug studies that require an Investigational New Drug (IND) application from the U.S. Food and Drug Administration (FDA). The rules and regulations in this area are a bit complex, but when the beginning investigator has worked his or her way through them once, they become understandable and even reasonable.

Exemptions

Clinical investigation with a drug that is already marketed in the United States is exempt from FDA requirements, if the investigation is not intended to be reported to the FDA to support a new indication for the drug (so that it can be marketed for a disorder for which it was not previously approved) or to support any change in the labeling of the drug.

This information was extracted from Title 21, CFR 312—Investigational Drug Application. Washington, DC, U.S. Food and Drug Administration, pp. 61–99.

It is also exempt if the study does not involve a new, non–FDA-approved route of administration or new dosage or use of the drug in a patient population that significantly increases the risks or decreases the acceptability of the risks associated with the drug. For example, if a drug that is used for the treatment of one disorder (e.g., depression) is being used in a study to treat a condition in which the risks of the use of the medication may be much higher (e.g., cardiac arrhythmias), even if the pharmaceutical firm is not involved and no attempt will be made to market the drug for that indication, the FDA still needs to be involved. If you have questions about this, you should contact the FDA for an opinion.

Costs

Although most researchers think of drug trials as being conducted "free of charge" to patients, IND regulations do allow a "sponsor" or "investigator" to charge for an investigational drug for treatment use under a treatment protocol, provided that 1) there is adequate enrollment in the ongoing clinical investigations under the IND, 2) the charging does not involve marketing, 3) the drug is not commercially advertised, and 4) the sponsor is already pursuing FDA approval. This would suggest that a drug nearing approval could be charged for in certain situations.

Phases

An IND may be submitted for one or more phases of investigation, although most clinical drug studies involving academic psychiatrists fall into phase III.

Phase I includes the initial use of an investigational drug in human subjects. Such subjects may include volunteer subjects or patients. These studies usually focus on metabolism, pharmacokinetics, side effects, and evidence of effectiveness.

Phase II studies include controlled trials to evaluate whether a drug is effective for a certain condition and to gain further experience regarding side effects and toxicity. Phase II trials are generally conducted in a small number of subjects and involve close monitoring.

Phase III studies include controlled trials further examining the effectiveness of a drug. Phase III studies of drugs intended for marketing often involve hundreds of subjects.

Control

FDA regulations allow the manufacturers of drugs to control to some extent the research done with them. This control is achieved through the specific IND requirements. An IND application needs to include certain technical information. If an investigator wants to use a compound in a research study, he or she can obtain authorization to refer to the manufacturer's IND, which includes the technical information necessary to support the study. If the manufacturer does not grant this permission, the investigator is nevertheless required to submit the same technical information supporting an IND, obtained on his or her own (which would be impossible for most investigators), or must be able to reference the necessary information in the literature (which is also highly unlikely). Therefore, a pharmaceutical firm, by granting or not granting permission to refer to its IND, is able to permit or prevent a clinical investigator's use of a drug for a non–FDA-approved indication if an IND is needed.

Applications

Specific IND forms are available from the FDA and require a great deal of specific information about the drug and the protocol. A specific protocol for each planned study needs to be included, and Phase II and III protocols need to be stipulated in great detail.

Information required includes the following:

- The objectives of the study
- The qualifications of all investigators
- The criteria for selection of subjects
- Study design
- Dosages
- Measurements
- Clinical laboratory procedures
- Detailed information concerning the chemistry, manufacturing, and control of the drug

Once an IND is in effect, it can be amended through submissions to the FDA.

IND Amendments and Safety Concerns

Sponsors are also required to report "information amendments" that are thought to be important for the IND, including new technical information about a drug and any report of discontinuation of an investigation. IND safety reports are also required. The sponsor has to notify the FDA and all participating investigators, using a written IND safety report, of any adverse experiences that are considered "both serious and unexpected." This should be done as soon as possible, "no later than 10 working days after the sponsor's initial receipt of the information." The sponsor is also required to notify the FDA by telephone of any unexpected "fatal or life-threatening experience associated with use of the drug in the clinical studies conducted under the IND," no later than 3 working days after receiving such information, with follow-up information in the form of a safety report to be submitted as soon as possible. Also, sponsors have to submit annual reports within 60 days of the anniversary date when the IND went into effect; the report must include a summary of the status of each study.

A special process allows a physician to obtain a *treatment protocol* or *treatment IND,* in which a non–FDA-approved drug can be used for a given patient if he or she has an illness that is "serious or immediately life-threatening" and for whom "no comparable or satisfactory alternative drug or therapy is available." Such use is unlikely to be approved before Phase II.

IND Approval

Relative to approval, an IND automatically goes into effect 30 days after submission unless the FDA notifies the sponsor that the investigation described in the IND is subject to a *clinical hold.* The FDA may request a clinical hold for several reasons. For example, the FDA may deem that the risks outlined in the protocol are unreasonable or that clinical investigators are not adequately qualified to conduct the studies. Often, the FDA requests fairly minor modifications in a protocol, such as pregnancy testing for female subjects.

The FDA may at any time terminate an IND, at which time the sponsor has to stop all clinical investigations. There are several grounds for termination, such as unreasonable risk to human subjects, problems with the manufacturing, deviations from the protocols, or evidence that the drug appears to be ineffective.

The FDA also has fairly strict guidelines on a number of other issues of relevance to such protocols, including selecting investigators ("qualified by training and experience as appropriate experts to investigate" the drug), proper control of the drug, and evidence that the study sites will conduct the protocol in compliance with the IND. The sponsor must provide each investigator with an *investigator brochure,* containing detailed information about the drug and the procedures in the protocol. These brochures (perhaps better described as large-metropolitan-area telephone books rather than brochures) need to be periodically updated by the sponsor, particularly relative to new data on adverse effects.

Monitoring

The sponsor must monitor the progress of all clinical investigations. If the sponsor determines that an investigational drug presents an "unreasonable and significant risk," the sponsor is supposed to discontinue such investigations and notify the FDA as well as all the involved Institutional Review Boards and investigators "as soon as possible and no later than 5 working days" after making such a determination. The FDA has the right to inspect all records or to request a sponsor to submit records.

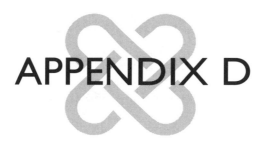

APPENDIX D

Scales and Questionnaires for the Diagnosis and Assessment of Psychiatric Disorders in Clinical Psychiatric Research

Diagnostic Interview Schedules

Schedule for Affective Disorders and Schizophrenia (SADS; Endicott and Spitzer 1978)

Features.   The SADS is designed to assess Research Diagnostic Criteria (RDC) and requires a trained interviewer knowledgeable about psychopathology. It generally takes 1–2 hours to administer.

Structured Clinical Interview for DSM-IV (SCID; First et al. 1997a, 1997b)

Features.   The SCID is designed to yield DSM diagnoses; the latest SCIDs assess for DSM-IV (American Psychiatric Association 1994). Different versions are available, depending on the population to be studied. The instrument should be used by trained raters knowledgeable about psychopathology.

Diagnostic Interview Schedule (DIS; Robins et al. 1979)

Features. The DIS was designed for epidemiological research and can be administered by nonclinicians who are carefully trained in its use. It was originally designed to assess Feighner criteria and can be used to score RDC. It takes 1–2 hours to administer.

Schizophrenia and Other Nonaffective Psychosis Scales

Brief Psychiatric Rating Scale (BPRS; Overall and Gorham 1962)

Features. The BPRS was designed for use in patients with schizophrenia and patients with other psychotic disorders. The most recent version has 18 items. Factor analysis identifies 5 subfactors: thought disorder, emotional withdrawal, agitation, anxiety-depression, and aggressiveness. The scale is widely used in pharmacological studies involving schizophrenic patients.

Positive and Negative Syndrome Scale (PANSS; Kay et al. 1986)

Features. The PANSS is a symptom severity scale designed to measure positive and negative symptoms. Each subscale has 7 items, and a general psychopathology scale includes 16 items.

Scale for the Assessment of Negative Symptoms (SANS; Andreasen 1982)

Features. The SANS includes 30 items, and the total score indicates severity.

Rating Scale for Emotional Blunting (Abrams and Taylor 1978)

Features. This 16-item scale is rated by psychiatrists following a clinical interview.

Depression Scales

Beck Depression Inventory
(BDI-I, BDI-II; Beck et al. 1961)

Features. The BDIs are 21-item self-administered scales measuring depression severity and commonly used in psychopharmacological trials.

Zung Self-Rating Depression Scale (Zung 1965)

Features. This 20-item self-rating scale is used to measure depression severity.

Montgomery-Åsberg Rating Scale for Depression
(Montgomery and Åsberg 1979)

Features. This observer-rated 10-item scale is used to measure depression severity.

Hamilton Rating Scale for Depression
(Ham-D; Hamilton 1960)

Features. The Ham-D is a clinician-rated instrument most commonly used in a 21-item form. It is one of the most widely used scales in psychopharmacological research in depression.

Mania Scales

Rating Scale for Mania (Young et al. 1978)

Features. This clinician-rated 11-item scale is used to measure the overall level of mania severity.

Manic-State Rating Scale (Blackburn et al. 1977)

Features. This observer-rated inventory can be used to measure change in manic state.

Obsessive-Compulsive Symptoms Scales

Yale-Brown Obsessive Compulsive Scale (Y-BOCS; Goodman et al. 1989a, 1989b)

Features. The Y-BOCS is a clinician-rated instrument. It can take an hour to administer in symptomatic patients. Sixteen items are rated on a 5-point scale, 10 of which are used to provide a final score. Areas of focus include interference, resistance, distress, control, and time spent on obsessions and compulsions.

Leyton Obsessional Inventory (Cooper 1970)

Features. This supervised card-sorting task includes 69 questions. It can be administered by a layperson.

Anxiety Scales

Hamilton Anxiety Scale (Ham-A; Hamilton 1959)

Features. The Ham-A is a clinician-rated 14-item instrument based on an interview. It is frequently used to measure response in psychopharmacological trials.

State-Trait Anxiety Inventory (Spielberger et al. 1970)

Features. This 40-item questionnaire is designed to measure both state and trait anxiety and is widely used in psychological research.

Taylor Manifest Anxiety Scale (Taylor 1953)

Features. This 50-item scale is designed to separate situational from nonsituational problems with anxiety. The Taylor Manifest Anxiety Scale correlates highly with the trait section of the State-Trait Anxiety Inventory.

Personality Disorders Assessment: Structured Clinical Interviews

Structured Clinical Interview for DSM-IV Axis II Personality Disorders (SCID-II; First et al. 1997b)

Features. The SCID-II is a clinician-administered semistructured interview used to diagnose the 11 DSM-IV Axis II personality disorders. Its design is unique in its primary goal of rapid clinical assessment of personality disorders without sacrificing reliability or validity. It can be used with a self-report questionnaire, which may shorten the overall interview time.

Personality Disorder Examination (PDE; Loranger et al. 1985)

Features. The PDE is a 126-item semistructured interview for use by experienced clinicians. It provides dimensional scores and diagnoses for each of the DSM-IV personality disorders. It also assesses domains of functioning (e.g., personal relationships), which can be converted into DSM-IV personality disorder diagnoses.

Structured Interview for DSM-IV Personality (SIDP-IV; Pfohl et al. 1997)

Features. The SIDP-IV is an interview organized into 10 sections for domains of behavior associated with personality disorders. It is administered by trained clinicians and covers all the DSM-IV personality disorder constructs.

Personality Disorders Assessment: Self-Report Questionnaires

Personality Diagnostic Questionnaire (PDQ-R; Hyler and Rieder 1987)

Features. The PDQ-R is a 162-item, true-false questionnaire that yields both dimensional scores and personality disorder diagnoses consistent with the DSM personality disorder criteria then in use. It also yields an impairment and distress score.

Millon Clinical Multiaxial Inventory—II (MCMI-II; Millon 1987)

Features. The MCMI-II is a 175-item self-report questionnaire that includes 13 scales designed to measure personality disorders. Eleven of the scales correspond to the DSM-III-R Axis II personality disorders. Scales are also included to assess self-defeating personality disorder and aggressive-sadistic personality disorder, diagnoses that had been proposed at that time.

Wisconsin Personality Disorders Inventory (WISPI; Klein et al. 1993)

Features. The WISPI is a 214-item self-report questionnaire that offers dimensional scores and categorical diagnoses of DSM-IV personality disorder constructs.

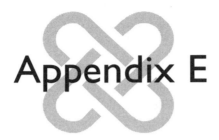

Appendix E

Web Sites: Resources for Research and Ethics

American Association of Bioethics
  http://www.med.umn.edu/aab/

Belmont Report (Ethical Principles and Guidelines)
  http://helix.nih.gov:8001/ohsr/mpa/belmont.phtml

Bioresearch Monitoring (FDA Program)
  http://www.fda.gov/ora/compliance_ref/bimo/default.html

CBER (Center for Biologics Evaluation and Research)
  http://www.fda/gov/cber/index.html

CDC (Centers for Disease Control and Prevention)
  http://www.cdc.gov/

CDER (Center for Drug Evaluation and Research)
  http://www.fda.gov/cder/

CFR (Code of Federal Regulations)
  http://www.access.gpo.gov/nara/cfr/cfr-table-search.html

Declaration of Helsinki (Biomedical Research Recommendations)
  http://www.etikkom.no/NEM/REK/declaration96.htm

DHHS (Department of Health and Human Services)
  http://www.os.dhhs.gov/

FDA (Food and Drug Administration)
http://www.fda.gov/fdahomepage.html

GPO (Government Printing Office)
http://www.access.gpo.gov/su_docs/

Guide to Good Clinical Practice
http://www.thompson.comtpg/food/clin/clintoc.html

MedWatch (FDA Medical Products Reporting)
http://www.fda.gov/medwatch/

NBAC (National Bioethics Advisory Commission)
http://www.bioethics.gov/

NHGRI (National Human Genome Research Institute)
http://www.nhgri.nih.gov/

NIH (National Institutes of Health)
http://www.nih.gov/

NSF (National Science Foundation)
http://www.nsf.gov/

Nuremberg Code (directives for human experimentation)
http://helix.nih.gov:8001/ohsr/nuremberg.phtml

OPRR (Office of Protection from Research Risks)
http://www.grants.nih.gov./grants/oprr/oprr.htm

ORI (Office of Research Integrity)
http://ori.dhhs.gov

PHS (Public Health Service)
http://phs.os.dhhs.gov/phs/phs.html

USDA (Department of Agriculture)
http://www.usda.gov/

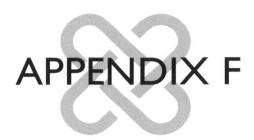

APPENDIX F

Contacts and Telephone Numbers at the National Institutes of Health (NIH)

Note. Several of the institutes listed were undergoing reorganization at the time of writing. Therefore, the contact information listed is accurate as of that time. For additional help with contact information, please call the numbers listed. For NIMH, you can also check the Web site for help: http://www.nimh.gov/about/locator_org.cfm.

National Institute on Alcohol Abuse and Alcoholism (NIAAA)

6000 Executive Boulevard, Willco Building
Bethesda, Maryland 20892-7003
(301) 443-3860
http://www.niaaa.nih.gov

Grants Management Officer and Grants Management Contracts

Ms. Linda Hilley
Deputy Chief, Grants Management Branch
Willco Building, Suite 504
(301) 443-0915

Staff:
Ms. Patricia Byrd
Mr. Edward Ellis
Ms. Deborah Hendry
Mr. Gene McGeehan
Ms. Judy Simons

Division of Clinical and Prevention Research
Dr. Richard Fuller
Director
Willco Building, Suite 505
(301) 443-1208

Program Contacts
Prevention Research Branch
Dr. Jan Howard
Chief
Willco Building, Suite 505
(301) 443-1677

Treatment Research Branch
Dr. Richard Fuller
Acting Chief
Willco Building, Suite 505
(301) 443-0633

Division of Basic Research
Dr. Sam Zakhari
Director
Willco Building, Suite 402
(301) 443-0799

Program Contacts
Biomedical Research Branch
Dr. Tom Kresina
Chief
Willco Building, Suite 402
(301) 443-4224

Neurosciences and Behavioral Research Branch
Dr. Antonio Noronha
Chief
Willco Building, Suite 402
(301) 443-4223

Division of Biometry and Epidemiology
Dr. Mary Dufour
Director
Willco Building, Suite 514
(301) 443-3851

Program Contacts

Biometry Branch
Dr. Bridget Grant
Chief
Willco Building, Suite 514
(301) 443-3306

Epidemiology Branch
Dr. Darryl Bertolucci
Acting Chief
Willco Building, Suite 514
(301) 443-4897

Scientific Review (program projects, centers, training, and careers)
Dr. Kenneth Warren
Director, Office of Scientific Affairs
Office of Scientific Affairs
Willco Building, Suite 409
(301) 443-5494

Dr. Mark Green
Chief, Extramural Project Review Branch
Willco Building, Suite 409
(301) 443-2860

Ms. Diane Miller
Chief, Scientific Communication Branch
Willco Building, Suite 409
(301) 443-3860

Information Contacts for Funding Status
Competing: Contact appropriate program staff
Noncompeting: Grants management contact listed on award notice
Administration of grants: Grants management contacted listed on award notice

National Institute on Drug Abuse (NIDA)

6000 Executive Boulevard, Willco Building
Bethesda, Maryland 20892-7003
(301) 443-3860
http://www.niaaa.nih.gov

Grants Management Officer

Dr. Gary Fleming
Chief, Grants Management Branch
(301) 443-6710

Program/Division Directors

Division of Epidemiology, Services and Prevention Research
Ms. Ann Blanken
Acting Director
(301) 443-6504

Division of Neuroscience and Behavioral Research
Dr. Karen Skinner
Acting Director
(301) 443-1887

Division of Treatment Research and Development
Dr. Frank Vocci
Director
(301) 443-6173

Center on AIDS and Other Medical Consequences
Dr. Henry Francis
Director
(301) 443-1801

Office of Extramural Program Review
Dr. Teresa Levitin
Director
(301) 443-2755

Office of Science Policy and Communications
Dr. Timothy Condon
Director
(301) 443-6036

SBIR Coordinator
Dr. Cathrine Sasek
Coordinator, Science Education Program
(301) 594-6312

Information Contacts for Funding Status
Competing: Name of program person assigned to application
Noncompeting: Grants management contact listed on award notice
Administration of grants: Grants management contact listed on award
notice

Payback and Trainee Appointment Forms
Dr. Jack Manischewitz
Grants Management Specialist
(301) 443-6710

National Institute of Mental Health (NIMH)

Note. *For all the addresses below at the Neuroscience Center, the city, state, and ZIP code are Bethesda, MD 20892. In addition, any address listed with a Mail Stop Code (MSC) must have a 9-digit ZIP code. The last 4-digit portion must correspond to the Mail Stop Code. See example below: MSC 9663 and Bethesda, MD 20892-9663.*

Neuroscience Center, Room 8184, MSC 9663
6001 Executive Boulevard
Bethesda, Maryland 20892-9663
(301) 443-4513
http://www.nimh.nih.gov

Grants Management Branch
Mrs. Diana Trunnell
Assistant Chief
Neuroscience Center, Room 6115, MSC 9605
(301) 443-2805

Program Contacts

Office of Special Populations
Mr. Sherman Ragland
Acting Director
Neuroscience Center, Room 8125, MSC 9659
(301) 443-2847

Office on AIDS
Dr. Ellen Stover
Director
Neuroscience Center, Room 6225, MSC 9621
(301) 443-9700

Office of Science Policy and Program Planning

Dr. Brent Stanfield
Director
Neuroscience Center, Room 8208, MSC 9667
(301) 443-4335

Division of Neuroscience and Basic Behavioral Science

Dr. Stephen Foote
Acting Director
Neuroscience Center, Room 7204, MSC 9645
(301) 443-3563

Behavioral Science Research Branch
Dr. Mary Ellen Oliveri
Chief
Neuroscience Center, Room 7220, MSC 9651
(301) 443-9400

Behavioral and Integrative Neuroscience Research Branch
Dr. Kevin Quinn
Acting Chief
Neuroscience Center, Room 7168, MSC 9637
(301) 443-1576

Clinical Neuroscience Research Branch
Dr. Steven Zalcman
Chief
Neuroscience Center, Room 7177, MSC 9639
(301) 443-1692

Genetics Research Branch
Dr. Steven Moldin
Chief
Neuroscience Center, Room 7189, MSC 9643
(301) 443-9869

Molecular and Cellular Neuroscience Research Branch
Dr. Linda Brady
Acting Chief
Neuroscience Center, Room 7185, MSC 9641
(301) 443-5288

Division of Services and Intervention Research

Dr. Grayson Norquist
Director
Neuroscience Center, Room 7117, MSC 9629
(301) 443-3266

Adult and Geriatric Treatment and Preventive Intervention Research Branch
Dr. Barry Lebowitz
Chief
Neuroscience Center, Room 7160, MSC 9635
(301) 443-1185

Child and Adolescent Treatment and Preventive Intervention Research Branch
Dr. Benedetto Vitiello
Chief
Neuroscience Center, Room 7149, MSC 9633
(301) 443-4283

Services Research and Clinical Epidemiology Branch
Dr. Grayson Norquist
Chief
Neuroscience Center, Room 7117, MSC 9631
(301) 443-3266

Division of Mental Disorders, Behavioral Research and AIDS

Dr. Ellen Stover
Director
Neuroscience Center, Room 6217, MSC 9621
(301) 443-9700

Adult Psychopathology and Prevention Research Branch
Dr. Bruce Cuthbert
Branch
Chief Neuroscience Center, Room 6186, MSC 6625
(301) 443-3728

Center for Mental Health Research on AIDS
Dr. Ellen Stover
Director
Neuroscience Center, Room 6225, MSC 9619
(301) 443-9700

Developmental Psychopathology and Prevention Research Branch
Dr. Doreen Koretz
Chief
Neuroscience Center, Room 6200, MSC 9617
(301) 443-5944

Health and Behavioral Science Research Branch
Dr. Peter Muehrer
Chief
Neuroscience Center, Room 6190, MSC 9615
(301) 443-4708

Division of Extramural Activities
Dr. Jane Steinberg
Acting Director
Neuroscience Center, Room 6154, MSC 9607
(301) 443-3367

Note. *The Division of Extramural Activities responds to review process questions; the research divisions respond to inquiries on science and the application process.*

Clinical Review Branch
Dr. Gerald Calderone
Scientific Review Administrator
Neuroscience Center, Room 6150, MSC 9608
(301) 443-1340

Neuroscience and Behavioral Science Review Branch
Dr. Laurence Stanford
Chief
Neuroscience Center, Room 6138, MSC 9606
(301) 443-1178

Freedom of Information Office
Ms. Marilyn Weeks
Public Affairs Specialist
Neuroscience Center, Room 8184, MSC 9663
(301) 443-4536

Public Affairs and Science Reports
Ms. Clarissa Wittenberg
Director, Office of Communications and Public Liaison
Neuroscience Center, Room 8184, MSC 9663
(301) 443-3600

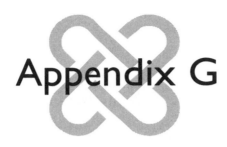

Appendix G

National Institutes of Health Grant Application Reviews

Various funding mechanisms are available through the National Institutes of Health (NIH). A great deal of information about these mechanisms, how grant applications are reviewed, and other valuable information for those seeking NIH funding are available on the Web at www.nih.gov. The data included in this appendix were obtained at that Web site. Beginning investigators are encouraged to become familiar with the Web site and the various types of information available there.

NIH Review Criteria

In considering the submission of grant applications, a very important document to keep in mind is the review criteria used by those on the review committees who will be seeing your application. They will be using these criteria in their decision about the merit of the application, and therefore aspiring grantees should bear the criteria in mind during preparation.

The following material has been excerpted from "Review Criteria for and Rating of Unsolicited Research Grant and Other Applications," *NIH Guide,* Volume 26, Number 22, June 27, 1997, P.T. 34 ("Review Criteria" 1997). This document went into effect for reviews conducted as of January/February 1998 (bold type is the authors').

Excerpts from "Review Criteria"

Background

As part of the ongoing effort to maintain high standards for peer review at the NIH, the Rating of Grant Applications (RGA) subcommittee of the NIH Committee on Improving Peer Review was charged with examining the process by which scientific review groups rate grant applications and with making recommendations to improve that process in light of scientific knowledge of measurement and decision making. The charge was in response to the perception that the review of grant applications needed to be refocused on the quality of the science and the impact it might have on the field, rather than on details of technique and methodology.

Reviewers will be instructed to: a) address the five review criteria below, and b) assign a single, global score for each scored application. The score should reflect the overall impact that the project could have on the field based on consideration of the five criteria, with the emphasis on each criterion varying from one application to another, depending on the nature of the application and its relative strengths.

The goals of NIH-supported research are to advance our understanding of biological systems, improve the control of disease, and enhance health. In the written comments reviewers will be asked to discuss the following aspects of the application in order to judge the likelihood that the proposed research will have a substantial impact on the pursuit of these goals. **Each of these criteria will be addressed and considered in assigning the overall score, weighting them as appropriate for each application. Note that the application does not need to be strong in all categories to be judged likely to have major scientific impact and thus deserve a high priority score.** For example, an investigator may propose to carry out important work that by its nature is not innovative but is essential to move a field forward.

1. **Significance: Does this study address an important problem? If the aims of the application are achieved, how will scientific knowledge be advanced? What will be the effect of these studies on the concepts or methods that drive this field?**

2. **Approach: Are the conceptual framework, design, methods, and analyses adequately developed, well-integrated, and appropriate to the aims of the project? Does the applicant acknowledge potential problem areas and consider alternative tactics?**

3. Innovation: Does the project employ novel concepts, approaches or method? Are the aims original and innovative? Does the project challenge existing paradigms or develop new methodologies or technologies?

4. Investigator: Is the investigator appropriately trained and well suited to carry out this work? Is the work proposed appropriate to the experience level of the principal investigator and other researchers (if any)?

5. Environment: Does the scientific environment in which the work will be done contribute to the probability of success? Do the proposed experiments take advantage of unique features of the scientific environment or employ useful collaborative arrangements? Is there evidence of institutional support?

While the review criteria are intended for use primarily with unsolicited research project applications to the extent reasonable, they will also form the basis of the review of solicited applications and non-research activities.

In addition to the above criteria, in accordance with NIH policy, all applications will also be reviewed with respect to the following:

- The adequacy of plans to include both genders, minorities, and their subgroups as appropriate for the scientific goals of the research. Plans for the recruitment and retention of subjects will also be evaluated.
- The reasonableness of the proposed budget and duration in relation to the proposed research.
- The adequacy of the proposed protection for humans, animals, or the environment, to the extent they may be adversely affected by the project proposed in the application.

(This ends the excerpts from the "Review Criteria" document.)

Submission Dates

Application receipt dates vary by type and are arranged over three cycles each year. In Table G–1, pay particular attention to the receipt dates for applications for New Research Grants (February 1, June 1, and October 1). Also notice that grant applications are first given a scientific merit review by a

Table G–1. Standard grant application receipt dates and review and award cycles

	Application receipt dates		
	Cycle I	Cycle II	Cycle III
Type of grant			
Individual National Research Service awards	January 10	May 10	September 10
All Academic Research Enhancement awards except those involving AIDS-related research	January 25	May 25	September 25
New Research grants, conferences, and Research Career awards; all Program Project and Center grants	February 1	June 1	October 1
Interactive Research Project grants	February 15	June 15	October 15
Competing continuation, supplemental, and revised grants	March 1	July 1	November 1
Individual National Research Service awards (standard)	April 5	August 5	December 5
All AIDS-related grants	May 1	September 1	January 2
Review and award schedule			
Scientific merit review	June–July	October–November	February–March
Advisory Council review	September–October	January–February	May–June
Earliest project start date	December	April	July

review group and that then the Advisory Council reviews the scores and makes final funding recommendations. It is important to note that a grant application submitted February 1 would have as the first *possible* start date the next December, but that because many grant applications will have to be resubmitted once or twice, the total process from first submission to funding can stretch for more than two years. Therefore, obtaining NIH funding is a long-term effort, and beginning investigators are advised to start the process as early as possible.

Number of Grants and Funding Amounts

Table G–2 shows the number of grant applications funded and the total amount in thousands of dollars awarded by each NIH component in 1998, the most recent data available. Much of the funding for research in clinical psychiatry comes from three institutes: the National Institute of Alcoholism and Alcohol Abuse (710 applications funded in 1998), the National Institute of Drug Abuse (1,480 applications funded in 1998), and the National Institute of Mental Health (2,076 applications funded in 1998).

Inclusion of Women and Minorities as Subjects

In the current funding situation, inclusion of women and minorities is of great importance. Investigators should familiarize themselves with the information available on the NIH Web site (see Appendix E) in this regard. NIH has established guidelines on the inclusion of women and minorities and their subpopulations in research involving human subjects, including clinical trials, supported by the NIH, as required in the NIH Revitalization Act of 1993. The guidelines describe the requirement for the inclusion of women and members of minority groups and their subpopulations in clinical research, including clinical trials, supported by NIH. These guidelines define clinical research as any NIH-supported biomedical and behavioral research involving human subjects.

The following text can serve as an introduction to NIH information on the NIH Web site. The text has been excerpted from "Notice of the NIH Guidelines on the Inclusion of Women and Minorities as Subjects in Clinical Research" ("Notice" 1994), published as a separate Part VIII in the Federal Register, March 28, 1994 (bold type is the authors').

Table G–2. NIH research grants by NIH component, fiscal year 1998 (in thousands of dollars)

NIH component	Number	Total amount
National Institute of Alcohol Abuse and Alcoholism (NIAAA)	710	180,213
National Institute on Aging (NIA)	1,508	414,518
National Institute of Allergy and Infectious Disease (NIAID)	3,455	974,645
National Institute of Arthritis and Musculoskeletal and Skin Diseases (NIAMS)	997	231,436
National Cancer Institute (NCI)	5,152	1,601,729
National Institute of Child Health and Development (NICHD)	1,841	485,608
National Institute of Drug Abuse (NIDA)	1,480	397,424
National Institute on Deafness and Other Communication Disorders (NIDCD)	727	161,968
National Institute of Diabetes and Digestive and Kidney Diseases (NIDDK)	3,081	725,197
National Institute of Dental Research (NIDR)	664	148,443
National Institute of Environmental Health and Sciences (NIEHS)	676	212,077
National Eye Institute (NEI)	1,290	296,203
National Institute of General Medical Services (NIGMS)	4,091	933,394
National Heart, Lung, and Blood Institute (NHLBI)	3,971	1,195,548
National Institute of Mental Health (NIMH)	2,076	558,972
National Institute of Neurological Disorders and Stroke (NINDS)	2,501	627,068
National Human Genome Research Institute (NHGRI)	236	161,991
National Center for Research Resources (NCRR)	741	416,601
Fogarty International Center (FIC)	153	6,845
National Library of Medicine (NLM)	82	15,907
National Institute of Nursing Research (NINR)	253	56,001

Excerpts from "Notice of the NIH Guidelines"

Since a primary aim of biomedical and behavioral research is to provide scientific evidence leading to a change in health policy or a standard of care, it is imperative to determine whether the intervention or therapy being studied affects women or men or members of minority groups and their subpopulations differently. To this end, the guidelines are intended to ensure that all

NIH-supported biomedical and behavioral research involving human subjects is carried out in a manner sufficient to elicit information about individuals of both genders and the diverse racial and ethnic groups and, in the case of clinical trials, to examine differential effects on such groups. Increased attention, therefore, must be given to gender, race, and ethnicity in earlier stages of research so that informed design of Phase III clinical trials can occur.

Policy

A. **Research Involving Human Subjects**

It is the policy of NIH that women and members of minority groups and their subpopulations must be included in all NIH-supported biomedical and behavioral research projects involving human subjects, unless a clear and compelling rationale and justification establishes to the satisfaction of the relevant Institute/Center (IC) director that inclusion is inappropriate with respect to the health of the subjects or the purpose of the research. Exclusion under other circumstances may be made by the Director, NIH, upon the recommendation of an IC director based on a compelling rationale and justification. Cost is not an acceptable reason for exclusion except when the study would duplicate data from other sources. **Women of childbearing potential should not be routinely excluded from participation in clinical research.** All NIH-supported biomedical and behavioral research involving human subjects is defined as clinical research. This policy applies to research subjects of all ages.

The inclusion of women and members of minority groups and their subpopulations must be addressed in developing a research design appropriate to the scientific objectives of the study. The research plan should describe the composition of the proposed study population in terms of gender and racial/ethnic group, and provide a rationale for selection of such subjects. The plan should contain a description of the proposed outreach programs for recruiting women and minorities as participants.

B. **Clinical Trials**

Under the statute, when a Phase III clinical trial is proposed, evidence must be reviewed to show whether or not clinically important gender or race/ethnicity differences in the intervention effect are to be expected. This evidence may include, but is not limited to, data derived from prior animal studies, clinical observations, metabolic studies, genetic studies, pharmacology studies, and observational, natural history, epidemiology, and other relevant studies.

As such, investigators must consider the following when planning a Phase III clinical trial for NIH support:

- If the data from prior studies strongly indicate the existence of significant differences of clinical or public health importance in intervention effect among subgroups (gender and/or racial/ethnic subgroups), the primary question(s) to be addressed by the proposed Phase III trial and the design of that trial must specifically accommodate this. For example, if men and women are thought to respond differently to an intervention, then the Phase III trial must be designed to answer two separate primary questions, one for men and the other for women, with adequate sample size for each.
- If the data from prior studies strongly support no significant differences of clinical or public health importance in intervention effect between subgroups, then gender or race/ethnicity will not be required as subject selection criteria. However, the inclusion of gender or racial/ethnic subgroups is still strongly encouraged.
- If the data from prior studies neither support nor negate strongly the existence of significant differences of clinical or public health importance in intervention effect between subgroups, then the Phase III trial will be required to include sufficient and appropriate entry of gender and racial/ethnic subgroups, so that valid analysis of the intervention effect in subgroups can be performed. However, the trial will not be required to provide high statistical power for each subgroup.

Cost is not an acceptable reason for exclusion of women and minorities from clinical trials.

C. Funding

NIH funding components will not award any grant, cooperative agreement, or contract and will not support any intramural project that does not comply with this policy. For research awards that are covered by this policy, awardees will report annually on enrollment of women and men, and on the race and ethnicity of research participants.

(This ends the excerpts from the "Notice of the NIH Guidelines" document.)

Types of NIH Support

The types of funding mechanisms available to investigators are quite numerous. Certain types of funding are of particular relevance to young investigators, particularly R03 grants (small research grants) and R01 grants (research projects). The NIH Web site, in addition to showing various grant funding opportunities, includes data on the likelihood of applications' being funded through these various mechanisms, funding rates by institution and state, and the variety of researchers conducting pilot research.

REFERENCES

Abrams R, Taylor MA: A rating scale for emotional blunting. Am J Psychiatry 135:225–229, 1978

American Psychiatric Association: Diagnostic and Statistical Manual of Mental Disorders, 4th Edition. Washington, DC, American Psychiatric Association, 1994

Anastasi A: Psychological Testing, 5th Edition. New York, Macmillan, 1982

Anderson C, Watson T: US drops Imanishi-Kari investigation; Baltimore withdraws cell retraction. Nature 358:177, 1992

Andreasen NC: Negative symptoms in schizophrenia. Arch Gen Psychiatry 39:784–788, 1982

Angell M: Editors and fraud. CBE Views 6:3–8, 1983

Angell M: Publish or perish: a proposal. Ann Intern Med 104:261–262, 1986

Angell M, Kassirer JP: The Ingelfinger Rule revisited. N Engl J Med 25:1371–1373, 1991

Annas GI, Grodin MA: The Nazi Doctors and the Nuremberg Code: Human Rights in Human Experimentation. New York, Oxford University Press, 1992

Appelbaum PS: Drug-free research in schizophrenia: an overview of the controversy. Review of Human Subject Research 18:1–5, 1996

Beck AT, Ward CH, Mendelson M, et al: An inventory for measuring depression. Arch Gen Psychiatry 4:561–571, 1961

Beecher HK: Ethics and clinical research. N Engl J Med 244:1354–1360, 1966

Beigel A, Murphy DL, Bunney WE: The Manic-State Rating Scale. Arch Gen Psychiatry 25:256–262, 1971

Blackburn IM, Loudon JB, Ashworth CM: A new scale for measuring mania. Psychol Med 7:453–458, 1977

Burdens of proof of misconduct (editorial). Nature 380:367, 1996

Burdock EI, Hardesty AS, Hakerem G, et al: Ward Behavior Inventory. New York, Springer, 1968

Campbell D, Stanley J: Experimental and Quasi-Experimental Designs for Research. Chicago, IL, Rand McNally College Publishing, 1963

Charney DS, Innis RB, Nestler EJ, et al: Increasing public trust and confidence in psychiatric research. Biol Psychiatry 46(1):1–2, 1999

Cook T, Campbell D: Quasi-Experimentation: Design and Analysis Issues for Field Settings. Chicago, IL, Rand McNally College Publishing, 1979

Cooper J: The Leyton Obsessional Inventory. Psychol Med 1:48–64, 1970

Cronbach LJ: Coefficient alpha and the internal structure of tests. Psychometrika 16:297–334, 1951

Dennis M, Ferguson B, Tyrer P: Rating instruments, in Research Methods in Psychiatry: A Beginner's Guide, 2nd Edition. Edited by Freeman C, Tyrer P. London, Gaskell/Royal College of Psychiatrists, 1992, pp 98–134

Derogatis LR, Cleary P: Confirmation of the dimensional structure of the SCL-90: a study in construct validation. J Clin Psychol 33:981–989, 1977

Draft Policy Statement on Industry-Supported Scientific and Educational Activities. Federal Register, November 27, 1992, pp 1–4

Elkin I, Parloff MB, Hadley SW, et al: NIMH Treatment of Depression Collaborative Research Program: background and research plan. Arch Gen Psychiatry 42: 305–316, 1985

Endicott J, Spitzer RL: A diagnostic interview: the Schedule for Affective Disorders and Schizophrenia. Arch Gen Psychiatry 35:837–844, 1978

FDA Information Sheets for Institutional Review Boards and Clinical Investigators. Rockville, MD, U.S. Food and Drug Administration, October 1995

Federal policy for the protection of human subjects: notices and rules. Federal Register, June 18, 1991, Part II, pp A4-1–A4-49

First MB, Spitzer RL, Gibbon M, et al: Structured Clinical Interview for DSM-IV Axis I. Washington, DC, American Psychiatric Association, 1997a

First MB, Gibbon M, Spitzer RL, et al: Structured Clinical Interview for DSM-IV Axis II Personality Disorders. Washington, DC, American Psychiatric Association, 1997b

Goldstein G, Hersen M: Historical perspectives, in Handbook of Psychological Assessment. Edited by Goldstein G, Hersen M. New York, Pergamon, 1990, pp 3–17

Goodman W, Price L, Rasmussen S: The Yale-Brown Obsessive Compulsive Scale: development, use and reliability. Arch Gen Psychiatry 46:1006–1011, 1989a

Goodman W, Price L, Rasmussen S, et al: The Yale-Brown Obsessive Compulsive Scale: validity. Arch Gen Psychiatry 46:1012–1016, 1989b

Green S, Lissitz R, Muliak S: Limitations of coefficient alpha as an index of test unidimensionality. Educational and Psychological Measurement 37:827–838, 1977

Guidelines for the study and evaluation of gender differences in the clinical evaluation of drugs. Federal Register 58, no. 139, July 22, 1993, p. 58 FR 39406

Hamilton M: The assessment of anxiety state by ratings. Br J Med Psychol 32:50–55, 1959

Hamilton M: A rating scale for depression. J Neurol Neurosurg Psychiatry 23:56–62, 1960

Hathaway SR, McKinley JC: The Minnesota Multiphasic Personality Inventory, Revised Edition. Minneapolis, University of Minnesota Press, 1943

Hays W: Statistics for the Social Sciences, 2nd Edition. New York, Holt, Rinehart & Winston, 1973

Hersen M, Bellack AS: Behavioral Assessment: A Practical Handbook, 2nd Edition. Elmsford, NY, Pergamon, 1981

Hirschfeld RMA, Klerman G, Clayton PJ, et al: Assessing personality: effects of depressive state on trait measurement. Am J Psychiatry 140:695–699, 1983

Honigfeld G, Klett C: The Nurses' Observation Scale for Inpatient Evaluation (NOSIE): a new scale for measuring improvement in schizophrenia. J Clin Psychol 21:65–71, 1965

Hyler S, Rieder R: PDQ-R Personality Questionnaire. New York, New York State Psychiatric Institute, 1987

International Committee of Medical Journal Editors: Uniform requirements for manuscripts submitted to biomedical journals. N Engl J Med 324:424–429, 1991

Kaiser J, Marshall E: Imanishi-Kari ruling slams ORI. Science 272:1864–1865, 1996

Kassirer JP, Angell M: On authorship and acknowledgments (editorial). N Engl J Med 325:1510–1512, 1991

Kassirer JP, Angell M: Financial conflicts of interest in biomedical research. N Engl J Med 329:570–571, 1993

Kay S, Opler L, Fiszebein A: The Positive and Negative Syndrome Scale (PANSS) Rating Manual. New York, Albert Einstein College of Medicine, Montefiore Medical Centre, 1986

Kazdin AE: Research design, in Clinical Psychology. New York: Allyn & Bacon, 1992

Kerlinger F: Foundations of Behavioral Research. New York, Holt, Rinehart & Winston, 1986

Kevles DJ: The assault on David Baltimore. The New Yorker, May 27, 1996

Klein MH, Benjamin LS, Rosenfeld R, et al: The Wisconsin Personality Disorders Inventory: development, reliability, and validity. J Personal Disord 7:285–303, 1993

Korenman SG, Shipp AC: Teaching the Responsible Conduct of Research Through a Case Study Approach: A Handbook for Instructors. Washington, DC, Association of American Medical Colleges, 1994

Kuder G, Richardson M: The theory of the estimation of test reliability. Psychometrika 2:151–160, 1937

Lanyon RI, Goldstein LD: Personality Assessment. New York, Wiley, 1971

Levine RJ: Ethics and Regulation of Clinical Research, 2nd Edition. New Haven, CT, Yale University Press, 1991, p x

Lewinsohn PM, Rosenbaum M: Recall of parental behavior by acute depressives, remitted depressives, and non-depressives. J Pers Soc Psychol 52:611–619, 1987

Loranger AW, Susman VL, Oldham JM, et al: Personality Disorder Examination (PDE): A Structured Interview for DSM-III-R Personality Disorders (Version May 15, 1985). White Plains, NY, The New York Hospital–Cornell Medical Center, Westchester Division, 1985

Lord F: On the statistical treatment of football numbers. Am Psychol 8:750–751, 1953

Maddox J: Making publication more respectable. Nature 369:353, 1994

Marwick C: Appeals board exonerates Baltimore, Imanishi-Kari. JAMA 276:266, 1996

Milestones in U.S. Food and Drug Law History. FDA Backgrounder, May 3, 1999. Web address: http://www.fda.gov/opacom/backgrounders/miles.html

Millon T: Manual for the MCMI-II. Minneapolis, MN, National Computer Systems, 1987

Montgomery SA, Åsberg M: A new depression scale designed to be sensitive to change. Br J Psychiatry 134:382–389, 1979

Morihisa JM, Rosse RB, Cross CD: Laboratory and other diagnostic tests in psychiatry, in Synopsis of Psychiatry. Edited by Hales RE, Yudofsky SC. Washington, DC, American Psychiatric Press, 1996, pp

National Bioethics Advisory Commission: Research Involving Persons With Mental Disorders That May Affect Decisionmaking Capacity, Vol 1: Report and Recommendations of the National Bioethics Advisory Commission, Rockville, MD. Rockville, MD, National Bioethics Advisory Commission, December 1998

National Commission for the Protection of Human Subjects of Biomedical and Behavioral Research: The Belmont Report: Ethical Principles and Guidelines for the Protection of Human Subjects of Research. Washington, DC: U.S. Department of Health, Education, and Welfare, 1979

Notice of the NIH guidelines on the inclusion of women and minorities as subjects in clinical research, Part VIII. Federal Register, March 28, 1994 (59 FR 14508–14513)

Nunnally J: Psychometric Theory. New York, McGraw-Hill, 1967

Oldham JM, Haimowitz S, Delano SJ: Protection of persons with mental disorders from research risk: a response to the report of the National Bioethics Advisory Commission. Arch Gen Psychiatry 56:688–693, 1999

Opinion; Imanishi-Kari Still in Limbo. Nature 368:1–2, 1994

Overall JE, Gorham DR: The Brief Psychiatric Rating Scale. Psychol Rep 10:799–812, 1962

Petersdorf RG: The pathogenesis of fraud in medical science. Ann Intern Med 104:252–254, 1986

Pfohl B, Blum N, Zimmerman M: Structured Interview for DSM-IV Personality (SIDP-IV). Washington, DC: American Psychiatric Press, 1997

Pocock SJ: Clinical Trials: A Practical Approach. New York, Wiley, 1983

Protecting Human Research Subjects: Institutional Review Board Guidebook. Office of Protection from Research Risks. Washington, DC, U.S. Government Printing Office, 1993

Review criteria for and rating of unsolicited research grant and other applications. NIH Guide 26(2), June 27, 1997, P.T. 34

Robins L, Helzer J, Croughan J, et al: The National Institute of Mental Health Diagnostic Interview. Rockville, MD, National Institute of Mental Health, 1979

Rothman DJ: Strangers at the Bedside: A History of How Law and Bioethics Transformed Medical Decision Making. New York, Basic Books, 1991

Schachman HK: What is misconduct in science? Science 261:148–149, 183, 1993

Seigel S: Nonparametric Statistics for the Behavioral Sciences. New York, McGraw-Hill, 1956

Spielberger CD, Gorsuch RL, Lushene RE: Manual to the State-Trait Anxiety Inventory. Palo Alto, CA, Consulting Psychologists Press, 1970

Spitzer R, Williams J, Gibbon M, et al: The Structured Clinical Interview for DSM-III-R, I: history, rationale and description. Arch Gen Psychiatry 49:624–629, 1992

Steele F: Clearing of researcher in Baltimore affair boasts demand for reforms. Nature 381:719–720, 1996

Stevens SS: Mathematics, measurement, and psychophysics, in Handbook of Experimental Psychology. Edited by Stevens SS. New York, Wiley, 1951, pp 1–49

Stone R: Federal panel recommends universities play bigger role (editorial). Science 267:449, 1995

Taylor JA: A personality scale of manifest anxiety. Journal of Abnormal and Social Psychology 48:285–290, 1953

Thomson KS: Scientific publishing: an embarrassment of riches. American Scientist 82:508–511, 1994

Uniform Requirements for Manuscripts Submitted to Biomedical Journals (special report). N Engl J Med 324:424–428, 1991

Wadman M: Hostile reception to US misconduct report. Nature 381:639, 1996

Wainer H, Thissen D: How is reliability related to the quality of test scores? What is the effect of local dependence on reliability? Educational Measurement: Issues and Practice 17:22–29, 1996

Weaver D, Reis MH, Albanese C, et al: Altered repertoire of endogenous immunoglobulin gene expression in transgenic mice containing a rearranged mu heavy chain gene. Cell 45:247–259, 1986

What to do about scientific misconduct (editorial). Nature 369:261–262, 1994

Wiens AN: Structured clinical interviews for adults, in Handbook of Psychological Assessment. Edited by Goldstein G, Hersen M. New York, Pergamon, 1990, pp 324–341

Woodward B: Challenges to human subject protections in US medical research. JAMA 282:1947–1952, 1999

Woolson R: Statistical Methods for the Analysis of Biomedical Data. New York, Wiley, 1987

Wright DT, Chew NS: Women and minorities in clinical research, I: women as subjects in clinical research. Applied Clinical Trials 5:44–54, 1996

Yager J, Burt VK: A survival guide for aspiring academic psychiatrists: personality attributes and opportunities for academic success. Academic Psychiatry 18:197–210, 1994

Young RC, Biggs JT, Ziegler VE, et al: A rating scale for mania: reliability, validity and sensitivity. Br J Psychiatry 133:429–435, 1978
Zimmerman M: Diagnosing personality disorders: a review of issues and research methods. Arch Gen Psychiatry 51:225–245, 1994
Zung WK: A self-rating depression scale. Arch Gen Psychiatry 12:53–70, 1965

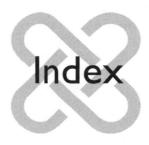

Index

Page numbers in **bold** type refer to tables or figures.